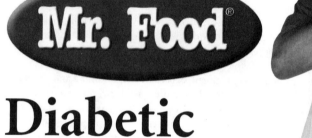

Diabetic Dinners in a Dash

More than 150 Fast & Fabulous Guilt-Free Recipes

By Art Ginsburg

Mr. Food

Featuring ADA Spokesperson

Nicole Johnson Baker

Miss America 1999

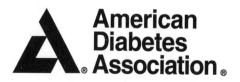

American Diabetes Association

Director, Book Publishing, John Fedor; *Managing Editor,* Abe Ogden; *Production Manager,* Melissa Sprott; *Printer,* Port City Press.

Mr. Food Managing Editor, Caryl Ginsburg Fantel; *Mr. Food Creative Director,* Howard Rosenthal; *Food Styling,* Howard Rosenthal and Patty Rosenthal; *Cover and Page Design,* Joe Peppi.

Printed in the United States of America
1 3 5 7 9 10 8 6 4 2

ADA titles may be purchased for business or promotional use or for special sales. To purchase this book in large quantities, or for custom editions of this book with your logo, contact Lee Romano Sequeira, Special Sales & Promotions, at the address below, or at LRomano@diabetes.org or 703-299-2046.

American Diabetes Association
1701 North Beauregard Street
Alexandria, VA 22311

Library of Congress Cataloging-in-Publication Data
Ginsburg, Art.
  Mr. Food diabetic dinners in a dash : more than 150 fast & fabulous guilt-free recipes / by Art Ginsburg ; featuring ADA spokesperson Nicole Johnson Baker.
      p. cm.
  Includes bibliographical references and index.
  ISBN 1-58040-241-0 (alk. paper)
  1. Diabetes--Diet therapy--Recipes. I. Title: Diabetic dinners in a dash. II. Title.

RC662.G546 2006
641.5'6314--dc22

2005034915

Dedicated to all the committed parents, spouses, children, and other caregivers who face the daily challenges of helping loved ones manage diabetes and its related complications. You are true heroes!

Contents

Foreword

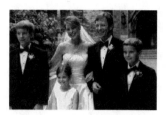 In the last few years, my life has changed dramatically. I went from being a single woman living on her own to being a married woman living in a house of six! Meal preparation now takes on a whole new meaning. There are six personalities to please and endless teenage appetites to whet. It is mind-boggling. Then, throw in diabetes, and you have a scenario that is often overwhelming and impossible to deal with.

Mr. Food Diabetic Dinners in a Dash to the rescue! This new cookbook solves many of my problems, including the teenage bottomless pits. It helps me come up with creative, delectable dishes to serve to my family. What fun we had experimenting and creating recipes to include along with the ones from Mr. Food. Even the kids got involved! By the way, getting involved is one of the key elements of this book. We want you and yours to enjoy the kitchen together, to learn about how foods affect your body, to understand what happens when you eat certain foods, and most important, to escape the trap of boring dinners.

Another benefit of these recipes is weight control. As we expand our horizons and as we become more engaged in food preparation and creative thinking, we become more satiated and therefore keep our weight in check. This is incredibly important to me, especially since I just had a baby. Diabetes during pregnancy left me somewhat in a bind in terms of food choices. Now, I am loving the experimenting and the ability to try new things as well as enjoy some old favorites.

Every recipe in this book is balanced in its approach to food groups. We don't advocate cutting any food category or food group from your meal plan; we advocate portion control and well-balanced variety. After more than 12 years with diabetes, I can tell you this is the only philosophy that works.

This book includes recipes designed to meet the needs of those with a variety of health concerns. If you are dealing with and/or trying to prevent conditions from diabetes to heart disease to celiac disease or even cancer, there is something in here for you. Food can either help or hurt you. We prefer the "help" and aim to give you choices that could improve your life. This is an unmatched resource full of ideas and, of course, unique inspiration and humor.

The point is to relax and enjoy your dinners. It *is* possible to have great dishes that are easy, low-key, and healthy. This is how we eat in the Baker house. We hope our favorites will inspire you to live better and manage your health in a smart way.

Sincerely,

Nicole Johnson Baker

Nicole Johnson Baker
Miss America 1999, Author and Diabetes Advocate

Preface

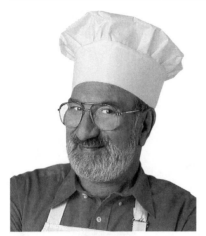

Art Ginsburg
Mr. Food

After writing my first two diabetes cookbooks, I was thrilled to hear from so many of you that my recipes had made mealtime not only easier for you but also much more enjoyable. Thank you for sharing your experiences with me!

Since then, you've asked me to write another book, one that focuses on great-tasting recipes that are really quick to prepare and satisfying for everybody in the family yet still fit a diabetes meal plan. I've tried to do that in this book, especially because I learned that the suggested meal plans for people with diabetes are similar to those for heart disease and cancer prevention.

In addition, I received many requests for recipes that would work for people with diabetes *and* celiac disease. Since celiac disease occurs in almost 1 in 10 children with diabetes, and 1 in 20 people with type 1 diabetes, the folks at the American Diabetes Association agreed with me on the importance of including recipes that would work for both types of meal plans. You'll see information regarding gluten-free items and options on the recipe pages that follow; see pages 10–13 for more information.

So, with all that in mind, it's important to know how to shop for the right ingredients to make delicious meals for your family that are healthy and help control diabetes. As you turn these pages, you'll find that my friend, diabetes advocate Nicole Johnson Baker, and I have come up with helpful tips that will have you dashing through the market making the right choices for nourishing meals that are fast and fabulous.

Speaking of dashing, we can't forget about the benefits of teaming simple exercise with our healthy eating lifestyle. There's more on that in here, too, so get ready to start today. My easy ideas are a guilt-free game plan for putting a super dinner on the table tonight and every night—one that's sure to have you and your family saying in a dash . . . **"OOH IT'S SO GOOD!!®"**

Mr. Food

Acknowledgments

It's never the efforts of one person that bring together a project of this magnitude. I am indebted to my terrific family and book production team (some of these people are part of both!) for making this book a reality. Howard Rosenthal is the creative force behind it all, while my daughter, Caryl Ginsburg Fantel, skillfully handles the editorial side for me.

Howard and Caryl adeptly manage the rest of our book production team, which starts with recipe coordinator Joe Peppi, test kitchen supervisor Patty Rosenthal, and recipe testers Diane Dolley and Terri Cahn. I have to thank my masterful recipe development team for their commitment and perseverance, since we demand that these recipes meet very strict taste and nutritional guidelines and, therefore, test our recipes many times to be sure they'll work for you every time.

While my kitchen staff was doing their job, the talented mother-daughter writing team of Helayne Rosenblum and Jerilyn Grunbaum was helping out on both the research and creative ends. And after taking a few books off, my daughter-in-law Carol Ginsburg returned to once again assist with the meticulous computer input of the completed recipes.

I appreciate the rest of my team just as much, including my son Steve Ginsburg, who heads the Mr. Food companies; my Executive Assistant, Debbi Friedman; Administrative Assistant, Jaime Gross; and Kitchen Assistant, Dio Gomez.

Working with Nicole Johnson Baker is always a joy. In our mutual quest to increase awareness of diabetes while improving the quality of life for people with diabetes, Nicole and I have developed a warm friendship that has strengthened over the years. Nicole's family has grown significantly since our last book, so I want to thank Scott and the kids, too, for suggesting that we include their family's favorite recipes in here. I also want to thank John Swanston for helping Nicole coordinate everything with us despite all our busy schedules.

It is a pleasure to be publishing another book with the American Diabetes Association. I appreciate the ongoing support of John Fedor, Director of Book Publishing, as well as the efforts of Managing Editor Abe Ogden. We also enjoy our continuing association with Lee Romano Sequeira, Director of Special Sales and Promotions.

Special thanks go to Karen L. R. Anderson, LCSW, RD, CDN, and Catherine (Katie) Marschilok, MSN, CDE, BC-ADM. Having a husband and three children with celiac disease, two of whom also have type 1 diabetes, Katie knows all too well about daily meal planning challenges. She was the first to share with me personal stories of dealing with the combination of diabetes and celiac, and she urged me to include recipes in my ADA books that would be suitable for both types of meal plans. Katie also steered us to Karen Anderson. Karen has celiac disease and, in her capacity as a registered dietitian, reviewed these recipes for us and deemed them either approved or not for gluten-free menu plans, or approved with gluten-free substitutions; you'll see these substitution options on the recipe pages. I applaud both of these women for working to increase awareness of celiac disease and diabetes and to improve the lives of those struggling with these diseases and their related issues.

Of course, I am ever grateful to my family, especially my wife, Ethel (the real "Mrs. Food"), who has shared so many wonderful Mr. Food moments and life experiences with me these many years.

Finally, I thank you, my loyal readers and fans who watch me every day on television, who come by to say hello when I make personal appearances, and who continue to write and request more quick-and-easy Mr. Food TV recipes and cookbooks. I delight in hearing of your progress in improving your health and well-being, and I wish you never-ending reasons to say . . .
"OOH IT'S SO GOOD!!®"

Introduction

Diagnosing and Managing Diabetes

Each year, the figures grow more alarming. Approximately 20.8 million people in the U.S. now have diabetes. Believe it or not, of that total, 6.2 million remain undiagnosed. I can't stress it enough—diabetes has been listed as the sixth leading cause of death in this country, yet with proper medication, diet, and exercise, it can be managed. Don't ignore the signs. Diabetes is best treated if caught early. If you think you or someone you know may be exhibiting symptoms of diabetes, see a physician immediately. Classic diabetes symptoms include the following:

• Frequent urination
• Excessive thirst
• Extreme hunger
• Unexplained weight loss
• Increased fatigue
• Irritability
• Blurred vision

If you've already been diagnosed, then there's a good chance that you've been advised by your physician and/or met with an RD (registered dietitian) who has analyzed your particular situation and offered practical ways for you to manage your diabetes.

We know that no single food will supply all the nutrients our bodies need, so variety is definitely still the "spice of life"—and there's still a lot you can eat. Under today's diabetes guidelines, it is refreshing to note that almost no food is forbidden. What's essential is a balance of foods and moderate portion sizes, along with exercise and medications, to manage blood sugar levels.

Unless you've been given different guidelines to follow, you should know these basic tips to help keep your blood glucose at a healthy level:

• Shop smart—that's where good eating habits start. Make a list and fill your cart with fresh foods in a wide variety of colors.
• Choose foods from a variety of food groups, limiting fats and sweets.
• Eat the same amount of food each day.
• Eat at about the same times each day.
• Take your medicines at the same times each day.
• Find a balance between food and physical activity, and exercise at the same times each day.

Taking Strides to Keep Healthy

Exercise is good for everyone, and it's especially helpful if you have diabetes. When you exercise, you will feel recharged physically and emotionally.

One of the best ways to maintain your health and help control diabetes is to walk. It's one of life's simplest pleasures that you can enjoy alone or with a companion—with no special equipment required. Plus, it's been documented that, through exercise, we just might be able to lower our risk of diabetes, heart attack, stroke, osteoporosis, and breast and colon cancers.

A stroll outdoors or even some time on a treadmill can be relaxing and beneficial. Of course, before starting a walking routine or any exercise program, check with your physician to make sure your heart and feet are in good shape. Once you get the okay, take the first step to good health—put on your walking shoes and reap the benefits in many ways:

Blood Glucose: Brisk walking, at a pace of 2 to 3 miles per hour, makes muscle cells more sensitive to insulin and helps lower blood glucose.

Heart Health: High blood pressure puts us at risk for heart disease, heart attack, and stroke. Brisk walking benefits the heart by lowering blood pressure. Walking can also lower LDL ("bad") cholesterol and triglycerides and raise HDL ("good") cholesterol. Improvement can occur in as little as a few weeks to three months.

Weight Control: Walking is extremely effective in helping with weight maintenance. If you are overweight and physically inactive, start slowly. Strive for a minimum of 30 minutes of walking every day, increasing the pace as you gain endurance.

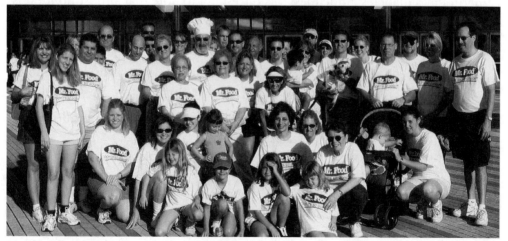

The Mr. Food team steps out annually to participate in raising awareness about diabetes as part of America's Walk for Diabetes. I'm so proud of my ever-growing team! Won't you join us in our efforts?

Energy Levels: Besides boosting your vitality and making you feel good, walking will make your muscles feel better and want to work. The more you walk, the more you'll build your endurance, and the easier it will get.

Mental Health: Studies have shown that regular exercise, including brisk walking, raises your heart rate. That generally results in the brain releasing serotonin, a chemical that helps elevate your mood and ease symptoms of depression and anxiety.

You see, as long as you've gotten your physician's clearance to exercise, there's no better time than today to start walking. And I recommend getting involved in America's Walk for Diabetes. Go to www.walk.diabetes.org for more information about America's Walk events in your area or to support the Mr. Food team in our fundraising efforts.

Size Matters

Portion size matters to everyone, but especially to people with diabetes and anyone adhering to a healthy diet. I've always said that moderation is key, with portion control being an important tool in managing diabetes. While portion sizes of things like bagels, muffins, and soft drinks have grown steadily in this country, so have restaurant portions of everything from steaks and French fries to pasta.

An important point to remember is that a "serving" is a standard amount set by the government, or sometimes by others, for recipes, cookbooks, or meal plans. A "portion" is how much food you choose to eat, whether in a restaurant, from a package, or in your own kitchen.

Fortunately, there are some easy ways to judge and control portion sizes:

• Read package labels carefully to find out what the serving size is. For instance, one muffin may actually equal two serving sizes, requiring us to cut that muffin in half to control our portions.

• When they're available, buy individual-serving sizes of packaged foods. Having nothing left over helps control the temptation to overeat.

• Give up your membership in the "Clean Plate Club." Try to leave a bit of each item on your plate at the end of your meal.

• Make your own sandwiches instead of picking them up from a deli. You can put together healthier lunches using whole-grain breads, lean meats, and extra vegetables.

- Serve yourself by making up your own plate in the kitchen, instead of at the dinner table. You'll reduce the temptation to indulge in seconds.

- When eating out, downsize your meal by ordering either an appetizer or lunch-sized version of a main dish as your meal.

- Also when eating out, as soon as your meal is served, set aside half of it and then enjoy the other half. This is a great way to guard against eating those inflated restaurant portions. Take home your second portion and enjoy it as a new meal the next day.

- Overindulging is commonplace at buffets, so either avoid them altogether or, if you must go, have a healthy snack at home first. At the buffet table, use a salad-sized plate to avoid piling too much on, and make light food choices.

- To prepare for those times when measuring tools aren't available, such as when you're dining out, learn to "eyeball" standard serving sizes, since it's important to stick to them. Measure out a controlled portion of your favorite meal the next time you have it, and remember what it looks like. Then you'll be able to recognize the proper serving size so you get it right. Here are some easy examples:

2 tablespoons peanut butter	=	golf ball
2 tablespoons salad dressing	=	ice cube
1 ounce bread	=	CD case
1 ounce cheese	=	lipstick tube or domino
3 ounces meat	=	playing card or palm of an average woman's hand
1/2 cup cooked vegetables	=	1 ear of corn, 3 broccoli spears, 6 asparagus spears, or 7 to 8 baby carrots
1 cup chopped fresh leafy greens	=	4 lettuce leaves
1 cup potatoes, rice or pasta	=	tennis ball or computer mouse
Medium apple or orange	=	baseball
1 standard bagel	=	hockey puck or 6-ounce can of tuna

Making Smart Food Choices

A trip to the supermarket can be daunting when you're trying to stick to healthy foods, whether or not you have diabetes. In our reading and on television, we're bombarded with survey results and statistics telling us what to avoid and what to overload on. All this information seems to make filling our shopping carts with the right choices only more confusing.

There are several food products that I receive regular questions about. The information in this section can help you make smart food choices.

Understanding Fats

Contrary to some people's understanding, our bodies need to take in a certain amount of fat. It aids in the absorption of vitamins A, D, E, and K and keeps our skin and hair healthy.

There are different types of fats, though, and it's important that we look more closely at which kinds of fats are good or bad for us and where they're found.

Monounsaturated fats and **polyunsaturated fats** are so-called "good" fats. They do not raise LDL ("bad") cholesterol levels and, when eaten in moderation, have significant health benefits. Sources of monounsaturated fats include avocados; sesame seeds; peanut butter; and peanut, olive, and canola oils. Sources of polyunsaturated fats include walnuts; pumpkin and sunflower seeds; corn, sunflower, and soybean oils; and fish.

Omega-3 fatty acids, also found in nuts and some fish (including salmon, sardines, and mackerel), are extremely healthful and are even thought to offer protection against heart disease.

The FDA Nutrition Facts Labels are now required to include information on any products that contain 0.5 grams or more of **trans fat** per serving. Trans fat is a liquid unsaturated fat that has been converted into a solid; this conversion process is called hydrogenation. Trans fat has been found to raise cholesterol—in particular, "bad cholesterol" LDL levels. This means that trans fat is linked to heart disease and stroke. Because it helps stabilize various foods, increasing their shelf life, it is found in items such as stick margarine, vegetable shortening, commercially prepared French fries and other fried foods, commercially prepared pastries and donuts, microwave popcorn, peanut butter, cake mixes, chips, and other foods.

In addition to trans fat, we need to be aware of and concerned about **saturated fat**, also known to raise cholesterol. Bakery products are a large source of saturated fat for many people, along with meat, milk, and milk products. That's why low-fat versions of these products are always preferable.

People with diabetes should limit their intake of trans and saturated fats, since having diabetes automatically increases the risk of heart disease and stroke. In fact, reducing the amount of trans and saturated fats in your diet is probably a good idea for everyone. Limiting calories from "bad" fat can also help you lose weight, especially when combined with an exercise program.

When checking food labels, combine the grams (g) of saturated fat and trans fat. Choose products with the lowest combined amount, as well as the lowest "Daily Value" percentage for cholesterol.

Fat-Cutting Cooking Tip

Use fat-free cooking sprays instead of butter, margarine, or oil for sautéing. Good choices are vegetable- and olive oil-based ones. Use a vegetable-based or refrigerated butter-flavored cooking spray for coating baking dishes.

Eggs and Egg Alternatives

Whole eggs contain a variety of beneficial nutrients, but they also contain things we don't want, such as high amounts of fat, calories, and cholesterol. By using an egg alternative, we get an even more nutritious product, since we eliminate 100% of the fat and cholesterol and more than half the calories. If that's not enough, egg alternatives contain greater amounts of folic acid, riboflavin, and vitamins A, B-12, D, and E.

The fact that egg alternatives are called "egg substitutes" leads people to believe that they're not real eggs, but they are. Most are 99% real egg—but only the egg white. Vitamins and other nutrients make up the remaining 1%, since we don't want to miss out on all those nutrients naturally found in egg yolks.

Not only are egg alternatives versatile and convenient, they're also pasteurized. This means that the health threats of salmonella and other diseases are normally eliminated if the eggs are consumed without having been cooked.

The next time you're at the supermarket, check out the egg alternatives, and give 'em a try.

Whole Grains

Though research is ongoing in many areas, there seems to be widespread agreement that the fiber content of whole grains has several health benefits.

A recent Harvard University study suggests that a diet that includes a variety of whole-grain foods may lower the risk of developing type 2 diabetes.

Researchers found that the whole-grain diet helped participants control their blood insulin levels. Tests also showed that the participants' bodies were better able to metabolize blood glucose, a step that keeps both insulin and glucose at healthier levels and may lower the risk of type 2 diabetes in those who do not yet have the disease.

Further research concluded that people who eat high-fiber foods have fewer heart attacks and strokes than those who don't. And fiber helps the digestive system by creating a "full" sensation, which is a big help with weight control.

When whole grains are refined into enriched white flour, most of their rich nutrients are lost. So although many whole-grain breads and pastas have a stronger taste than their refined-grain counterparts, with the right spreads and sauces we can enjoy them as healthier options.

What to look for when shopping:

• Whole-grain foods will list the grain—whole wheat, oats, rye—as the first ingredient on the food label.

• Look for whole-wheat pasta or one that is 50/50: half whole-wheat and half white flour.

• Choose cereals that are all of these: whole grain, high in fiber, and low in sugar.

Forget the white rice and white bread! Choose brown rice or whole-grain bulgur and breads with labels that contain the words "whole grain" or "whole wheat." And just because a bread is dark in color doesn't automatically mean that it's made from whole wheat; check the label.

Don't let the name of a product confuse you, either. If it states "made with whole wheat," "made with whole grain," "cracked wheat," "wheat flour," "enriched wheat flour," or "multi-grain," it is usually made with white flour or another refined grain, with only a small amount of whole wheat added.

Milk and Dairy Products

Milk and dairy products are a super source of calcium and should be included in a diabetes meal plan and any other healthy diet. However, according to the American Diabetes Association, it's important to keep your intake of saturated fat low, because it's been found to raise cholesterol levels, increasing the chances of developing heart disease.

Dairy products that contain saturated fat include full-fat cheese, cream, ice cream, whole milk, 2% milk, and sour cream.

Better choices:

Nonfat or low-fat yogurt, milk, and cheese are all excellent sources of calcium. Take advantage of the wide availability of light and reduced-fat cheese. Try different ones until you find the products you like best.

Many soy milks are also fortified with calcium, making them a good option if you are lactose intolerant or simply do not care for milk products. And if you must have your coffee light, use skim milk.

Traditional Dairy Products	Reduced-Fat Substitutions
Sour cream	Low-fat sour cream; low-fat or nonfat yogurt
Half-and-half	Fat-free half-and-half
American, Cheddar, Colby, Edam, or Swiss cheese	Reduced-fat and part-skim cheese with 5 grams of fat or less per ounce
Cottage cheese	1% low-fat cottage cheese
Cream cheese	Light cream cheese; 1/3-less-fat cream cheese
Ricotta cheese	Part-skim ricotta cheese
Milk, whole or 2%	Fat-free milk; low-fat (1%) milk
Ice cream	Fat-free or low-fat frozen yogurt; fat-free or low-fat ice cream; sherbet; sorbet

Cheesy Tips

You can use less of sharp or strong cheeses like Romano and feta because they have a more intense flavor than other types of cheese. Sometimes you can simply use less than the traditional amount of a "regular" full-fat cheese and still get the taste you enjoy.

Why Sugar Is Okay

The good news is that being diagnosed with diabetes doesn't mean sacrificing sweets! As you'll see in the American Diabetes Association–approved recipes in all my diabetic cookbooks, people with diabetes can use sugar, eat desserts, and still keep their blood glucose levels in their target range.

Research has shown that sugar has the same effect on blood glucose levels as other carbohydrates, such as breads and potatoes. Calorie for calorie, sugar raises blood glucose about the same amount as other carbohydrates.

Experts agree that, if you have diabetes, you can eat foods with sugar as long as you work them into your meal plan as you would any other carbohydrate-containing food; sugar is not a "free food" by any means. It's important that you make good choices about which carbohydrates to incorporate into your meal plan; ones that offer nutritious benefits, rather than "empty calories" (as is the case with sugar), are preferable.

Low- and no-calorie sweeteners are still an option for sweetening your foods and beverages. There are many options that the Food and Drug Administration (FDA) has approved for use in lieu of sugar. Discuss the choices with your physician and/or registered dietitian so that you can make the best decisions for your situation.

Shaking the Salt Habit

Diabetes increases your risk for high blood pressure. High levels of sodium (salt) in your diet can further increase that risk. So what can you do to add flavor to your recipes without turning to the salt shaker? Choose your favorites from these ideas and add them to your shopping list.

Herbs and Spices

Fresh or dried herbs and spices are must-haves for improving the natural flavors in food without using salt. Wait 'til you taste the excitement when you add:

• Assorted spice blends
• Basil
• Chili powder
• Cinnamon
• Cloves
• Cumin
• Curry powder
• Ginger
• Mint
• Nutmeg
• Oregano
• Parsley
• Thyme

Oils and Vinegars

For dressing salads, cooking, and basting, these add a healthy, guilt-free zip:

- Bottled reduced-fat Italian dressing
- Olive oil
- Sesame oil
- Flavored vinegars—there's red wine, white wine, balsamic, champagne, raspberry, sherry, and more!

Spreads and Sauces

East meets West when we put an international spin on our favorite recipes with one of these flavor enhancers. Each makes a great base for endless sauces, marinades, dressings, and dips:

- Dijon mustard
- Low-sodium soy sauce
- Salsa

Diabetes and Secondary Diseases

Unfortunately, there are many complications associated with diabetes. People with diabetes are at greater risk of developing heart disease, stroke, high blood pressure, blindness, kidney and nervous system diseases, dental disease, pregnancy complications, and more.

Don't be discouraged! There are things you can do to lower your risk of developing diabetes-related problems:

- Exercise daily.
- Maintain a healthy weight.
- Eat less fat and sodium.
- Eat more fiber: choose whole grains, fruit, vegetables, and beans.
- Quit smoking—seek assistance if necessary.
- Take medications as prescribed.
- Speak to your doctor about taking aspirin.
- Take the A1C test to measure your average blood glucose.
- Check your blood pressure regularly.
- Know your cholesterol numbers and keep them in the target ranges.

Diabetes and Celiac Disease

People with type 1 diabetes are also at greater risk for developing celiac disease, a chronic gluten-sensitive digestive disorder. Celiac disease can manifest itself at any age and cannot be outgrown. In individuals with celiac disease, exposure to gluten causes damage to the small intestine.

Symptoms of celiac disease include:

• Abdominal cramps, bloating, gas
• Anemia
• Bone pain
• Depression or irritability
• Early osteoporosis
• Fatigue, lack of energy
• Growth failure in children
• Heartburn
• IBS (Irritable Bowel Syndrome)
• Infertility or multiple miscarriages
• Lactose intolerance
• Neuropathy (tingling of the hands and feet)
• Unexplained weight loss

Gluten is a protein that is present in wheat, including durum, semolina, kamut, and spelt; rye; barley; triticale; and some oats. Since gluten ingestion can trigger painful gastrointestinal symptoms and poses serious health risks to people with celiac, a gluten-free lifestyle must be maintained.

A balanced diet is important to provide the nutrients everybody needs, so people with celiac disease should work with a physician and/or registered dietitian to prepare a meal plan that emphasizes complex carbohydrates (brown rice, legumes, fruit, vegetables) and a moderate intake of dairy and meat.

With celiac, not only must you avoid products that include wheat, rye, barley, and certain oats, but you must also read labels and be aware of possible hidden sources of gluten, such as these, in your foods and other everyday products*:

• Malt, malt flavoring, and malt vinegar, which are derived from barley
• Anything referred to as "binders," "fillers," or "extenders"
• Dairy substitutes: anything, such as rice or soy milk, that contains barley or malt flavoring
• Anything called "natural flavoring"
• Starch or modified food starch, used in many commercial dried spices: may contain wheat or barley (read all labels and/or check with the manufacturers)
• HPP (hydrolyzed plant protein) and HVP (hydrolyzed vegetable protein): may use wheat, rye, barley, or oats as protein sources

*This is by no means a complete listing of foods and products that contain gluten.

These common products may also contain gluten*:

• Licorice: contains wheat
• Prepared cake frosting: may contain wheat starch
• Processed cheeses, including cheese slices and other forms: may contain modified food starch
• Soy sauce: may contain wheat or barley
• Play-Doh: contains wheat
• Stamps and envelopes: the glue may contain wheat
• Lipstick: may contain wheat starch as a filler or dispensing agent

*This is by no means a complete listing of foods and products that contain gluten.

It is vital for a person with celiac disease to carefully scrutinize the labels of all products that could be ingested. Lipstick is a perfect example of something you might not think of as containing gluten, but it does if it contains wheat starch as a filler or dispensing agent.

If you suspect that you or someone you know may have celiac disease, consult your physician as soon as possible. There is no cure, but there are ways to control it instead of letting it control you. (See "General Recipe Notes," page 13.)

Karen L. R. Anderson, the Registered Dietitian and nutrition counselor who assisted with gluten-free options for the recipes contained here, has this to say about living with celiac disease:

"As a dietitian and also one who lives with celiac, I try to stay positive, and I coach patients in my practice to do the same. To help those with celiac live well and happy on a gluten-free meal plan, I encourage them to focus on what CAN be eaten safely, and on the delicious possibilities out there. Individuals living with celiac know all too well the meaning of the word 'diet' and the concept of restriction, desperately craving what I call 'freedom of food choice.' With chefs and dietitians who are knowledgeable about and sensitive to gluten-free eating working together, freedom and satisfaction in eating are possible again . . . and the plate is no longer empty! It's wonderful!"

Karen, I couldn't have said it better!

General Recipe Notes

Since it is estimated that 1 in 20 people with type 1 diabetes also have celiac disease, we have added something new—gluten-free options—on our recipe pages. If a recipe has been designated as gluten-free, then we've put "Thumbs up for gluten-free meal plans!" on its page. If a recipe is NOT gluten-free as presented, but could be easily adapted, then we've included information on what products to check and substitution options, if appropriate. And if it would be complicated or impossible to convert a recipe to be gluten-free, then there is no indication or information about celiac on its page.

Packaged food sizes may vary by brand. Generally, the sizes indicated in these recipes are average sizes. If you can't find the exact package size listed in the ingredients, whatever package is closest in size will usually work in the recipe; experiment with different brands until you're satisfied, but please remember that using different products and/or package sizes may alter the recipe's nutritional analysis.

Unless otherwise specified, onions and other produce items called for in these recipes should be medium- or "average"-sized.

As I mention throughout this book, always use the lightest ingredients possible. And just because a product's name includes the word "light," doesn't necessarily make it so. You need to read and know what you're looking for on package labels. It's the best way to truly start lightening up your diet.

Appetizers

Zippy Mango Salsa

Serving Size: 1/4 cup; Total Servings: 12

2 large very ripe mangos, diced

1/2 medium green bell pepper, diced

1/2 medium red bell pepper, diced

1/2 small sweet onion, diced

2 tablespoons finely chopped fresh parsley

1/4 teaspoon hot pepper sauce*

1/4 teaspoon ground cumin*

1 In a medium bowl, combine all the ingredients; mix well.

2 Cover and chill for at least one hour before serving.

---

*To make this a gluten-free recipe, avoid hot pepper sauce with malt flavoring added, and use seasoning with no added starch from a gluten-containing source.

Exchanges
1/2 Fruit

Calories	35
Calories from Fat	2
Total Fat	0 g
Saturated Fat	0.0 g
Cholesterol	0 mg
Sodium	2 mg
Total Carbohydrate	9 g
Dietary Fiber	1 g
Sugars	7 g
Protein	0 g

"When looking for flavorful dishes that'll fit into your diabetes meal plan, you can't go wrong with salsas. Even though fruit contains carbohydrates, which can raise blood glucose levels, it's still important to keep it in your meal plan. Remember, it's mainly about portion control and balance. Try serving this salsa with low-fat tortilla chips at your next gathering, or use it to top fish or chicken dishes. It's super-fast and so versatile!"

Sun-Dried Tomato Pesto Dip

Serving Size: 1/4 cup; Total Servings: 16

Nonstick cooking spray*

2 packages (8 ounces each) fat-free cream cheese, softened

1/2 cup plus 1 tablespoon grated real Parmesan cheese, divided

1/3 cup light mayonnaise

2 tablespoons fresh lemon juice

1 teaspoon garlic powder*

1/2 teaspoon onion powder*

1/2 cup (approximately 10) sun-dried tomatoes, reconstituted and chopped (see Preparation Tip)

1/2 cup walnuts, toasted

1/3 cup packed fresh basil leaves

---

*To make this a gluten-free recipe, use seasonings with no added starch from a gluten-containing source and nonstick cooking spray with no flour added.

1 Preheat the oven to 350°F. Coat a 9-inch pie plate with nonstick cooking spray.

2 In a medium bowl, beat the cream cheese, 1/2 cup Parmesan cheese, mayonnaise, lemon juice, garlic powder, and onion powder until well blended.

3 In a blender or food processor, combine the sun-dried tomatoes, walnuts, and basil; process until finely chopped.

4 Add the tomato mixture to the cream cheese mixture; mix well then spoon into the pie plate. Sprinkle the remaining 1 tablespoon Parmesan cheese over the top.

5 Bake for 25 to 30 minutes, or until heated through. Serve at once.

Exchanges
1 Very Lean Meat
1 Fat

Calories 86
 Calories from Fat . . . 46
Total Fat . . . . 5 g
 Saturated Fat . . . . . . 1.1 g
Cholesterol . . . . 8 mg
Sodium . . . . 221 mg
Total Carbohydrate . . . . 4 g
 Dietary Fiber . . . . 1 g
 Sugars . . . . 2 g
Protein . . . . 6 g

Preparation Tip

To reconstitute sun-dried tomatoes, simply place them in a bowl, pour 1 cup boiling water over them, let sit for 5 minutes then drain. They'll plump right up.

South-of-the-Border Bean Dip

Serving Size: 1/4 cup; Total Servings: 14

2 cans (15-1/2 ounces each) pinto beans, rinsed and drained, divided

1 cup salsa, divided (see Options)

1 teaspoon canola oil

1 medium-sized onion, finely chopped

1 medium-sized green bell pepper, finely chopped

3 garlic cloves, minced

1 tablespoon dried cilantro*

2 teaspoons ground cumin*

3/4 teaspoon salt

1/2 cup (2 ounces) shredded Cheddar cheese

1 medium-sized tomato, chopped

1 In a blender or food processor, combine 1 can of beans and 1/4 cup salsa; blend or process until smooth.

2 In a large nonstick skillet, heat the oil over medium heat and sauté the onion, bell pepper, and garlic for 5 to 7 minutes, or until tender. Add the bean mixture, cilantro, cumin, salt, and the remaining can of beans and 3/4 cup salsa; mix well. Bring to a boil, reduce the heat to low, and simmer for 5 minutes, stirring frequently.

3 Pour the mixture into a shallow serving dish, top with Cheddar cheese and tomato, and serve warm.

*To make this a gluten-free recipe, use seasonings with no added starch from a gluten-containing source.

Exchanges

1 Starch

Calories	93
Calories from Fat	18
Total Fat	2 g
Saturated Fat	0.9 g
Cholesterol	4 mg
Sodium	322 mg
Total Carbohydrate	15 g
Dietary Fiber	4 g
Sugars	3 g
Protein	5 g

Options

Whether you're feeling hot-hot-hot or mild and mellow, this crowd-pleaser can be as mild or as spicy as you like. Just use your preferred intensity of salsa and serve with a variety of dippers like low-fat tortilla chips and flat bread— it's up to you!

Fresh Spinach Dip

Serving Size: 1/4 cup; Total Servings: 8

4 cups packed fresh spinach leaves

1/2 cup (2 ounces) crumbled reduced-fat real feta cheese

2 scallions, sliced

1/2 cup low-fat cottage cheese

1/4 cup light mayonnaise

1 tablespoon prepared horseradish

1 tablespoon chopped fresh dill

1 teaspoon fresh lemon juice

1/4 teaspoon salt

1/4 teaspoon black pepper

1 In a food processor or blender, blend all the ingredients until the mixture is smooth, scraping down the sides of the bowl as needed.

Thumbs-up for gluten-free meal plans!

Exchanges
1 Lean Meat

Calories 57
 Calories from Fat . . . 34
Total Fat . . . . 4 g
 Saturated Fat . . . . . . 1.2 g
Cholesterol . . . . 6 mg
Sodium . . . . 323 mg
Total Carbohydrate . . . . 2 g
 Dietary Fiber . . . . 1 g
 Sugars . . . . 1 g
Protein . . . . 4 g

"This great-tasting dip is a cinch to whip up when company drops by. Serve it with fresh vegetables for delicious, nutritious dipping that everybody can enjoy."

Roasted Red Pepper Hummus

Serving Size: 1/4 cup; Total Servings: 14

2 cans (15 ounces each) garbanzo beans (chickpeas), rinsed and drained, with 1/3 cup liquid reserved

1 jar (12 ounces) roasted red peppers, drained

3 garlic cloves

2 tablespoons fresh lemon juice

2 tablespoons olive oil

1 teaspoon ground cumin*

1 teaspoon salt

1 In a food processor, combine all the ingredients, including the reserved garbanzo bean liquid. Process until the mixture is smooth and no lumps remain, scraping down the sides of the bowl as needed.

2 Serve immediately, or cover and chill until ready to use.

*To make this a gluten-free recipe, use seasoning with no added starch from a gluten-containing source.

Exchanges

1 Starch

Calories	83
Calories from Fat . . .	28
Total Fat	3 g
Saturated Fat	0.4 g
Cholesterol	0 mg
Sodium	281 mg
Total Carbohydrate . . .	11 g
Dietary Fiber	3 g
Sugars	3 g
Protein	4 g

"Did you know that beans are high on the food pyramid as a 'beaneficial' source of fiber? Unlike other sources of carbohydrates, beans have been shown to produce low blood glucose response . . . so give this rich and creamy spread a try. It's as easy as 1-2-3, and it beats those store-bought versions by a mile."

Parmesan Pesto Pita Wedges

Serving Size: 6 triangles; Total Servings: 16

1/4 cup prepared pesto sauce

6 six-inch whole wheat pita breads, split

2 tablespoons freshly grated real Parmesan cheese

1 Preheat the oven to 350°F.

2 Spread 1 teaspoon pesto sauce on the smooth outer side of each pita half. Sprinkle each with 1/2 teaspoon Parmesan cheese. Cut each pita half into 8 equal wedges. Place in a single layer on large, rimmed baking sheets.

3 Bake for 8 to 10 minutes, or until crisp and golden. Serve immediately, or store in an airtight container until ready to serve.

Exchanges

1 Starch

Calories 69
  Calories from Fat . . . 18
Total Fat . . . . 2 g
  Saturated Fat . . . . . . 0.4 g
Cholesterol . . . . 1 mg
Sodium . . . . 74 mg
Total Carbohydrate . . . 12 g
  Dietary Fiber . . . . 1 g
  Sugars . . . . 1 g
Protein . . . . 3 g

"This traditional Middle Eastern flat bread makes a smart alternative to potato chips and heavier breads, because it's low in calories and carbohydrates. At my house we top pita wedges with practically everything, and with slices of grilled chicken breast or shrimp they make a hearty party appetizer or snack. Oh yes, since they're so easy to prepare, it's a fun way to get the kids to help out in the kitchen!"

Veggie-Stuffed Mushrooms

Serving Size: 2 mushrooms; Total Servings: 6

12 large mushrooms (about 3/4 pound)

1 tablespoon olive oil

2 small zucchini, shredded (about 1/2 pound)

1/2 small onion, finely chopped

1/2 red bell pepper, finely chopped

1/4 cup plain bread crumbs*

1/2 teaspoon garlic powder*

1/4 teaspoon salt

1/4 teaspoon black pepper

*To make this a gluten-free recipe, use a gluten-free bread crumb product and seasonings with no added starch from a gluten-containing source.

1 Preheat the oven to 350°F.

2 Remove the mushroom stems from the caps; finely chop the stems.

3 In a large skillet, heat the oil over medium heat. Add the mushroom stems, zucchini, onion, and bell pepper. Sauté the vegetables until tender, about 5 minutes. Add the bread crumbs, garlic powder, salt, and black pepper.

4 Stuff each mushroom cap with the vegetable mixture and place on a large, ungreased, rimmed baking sheet. Bake for 20 to 25 minutes or until the mushrooms are tender and heated through. Serve immediately.

Exchanges
1 Vegetable
1/2 Fat

Calories 65
  Calories from Fat . . . 26
Total Fat . . . . 3 g
  Saturated Fat . . . . . . 0.4 g
Cholesterol . . . . 0 mg
Sodium . . . . 136 mg
Total Carbohydrate . . . . 9 g
  Dietary Fiber . . . . 2 g
  Sugars . . . . 3 g
Protein . . . . 2 g

"This colorful starter welcomes almost any veggie you have on hand and proves that we eat with our eyes! Sprinkle these mushrooms with a bit of grated Parmesan cheese just before serving and watch how fast the gang digs in!"

Mini Margherita Pizza

Serving Size: 2 wedges; Total Servings: 16

4 eight-inch flour tortillas*

Nonstick cooking spray*

1/4 teaspoon dried oregano*

1/4 teaspoon garlic powder*

3 medium plum tomatoes, thinly sliced (about 3/4 pound)

2 tablespoons chopped fresh basil leaves

1/2 cup (2 ounces) shredded real mozzarella cheese

---

*To make this recipe gluten-free, use corn-flour tortillas, nonstick cooking spray with no flour added, and seasonings with no added starch from a gluten-containing source.

1 Preheat the oven to 350°F.

2 Lightly spray both sides of the tortillas with cooking spray and place on rimmed baking sheets. Bake for 5 to 6 minutes per side, or until crisp. Remove from the oven and sprinkle with oregano and garlic powder.

3 Layer the tortillas with tomato slices, basil, and mozzarella cheese. Return to the oven and bake for 5 to 6 minutes, or until the cheese is melted. Cut each tortilla into 8 wedges, and serve.

Exchanges
1/2 Starch

Calories 50
  Calories from Fat . . . 15
Total Fat . . . . 2 g
  Saturated Fat . . . . . . 0.7 g
Cholesterol . . . . 3 mg
Sodium . . . . 87 mg
Total Carbohydrate . . . . 7 g
  Dietary Fiber . . . . 1 g
  Sugars . . . . 1 g
Protein . . . . 2 g

"These mini pizzas are a terrific addition to any gathering since they go together so easily and cook up in less time than it takes to have pizza delivered!"

Lemon-Dijon Chicken Skewers

Serving Size: 3 strips; Total Servings: 8

1-1/2 pounds boneless, skinless chicken breast, cut into 24 strips

24 ten-inch skewers

1/4 cup fresh lemon juice

2 tablespoons Dijon mustard

1 tablespoon canola oil

2 teaspoons chopped fresh dill

1 teaspoon grated lemon peel

1/4 teaspoon salt

1/4 teaspoon black pepper

1 Preheat the grill to medium heat. If using wooden skewers, soak them in water for 15 minutes.

2 Thread each chicken strip onto a skewer.

3 In a small bowl, combine the remaining ingredients; mix well. Dip chicken skewers into lemon-Dijon sauce, coating completely.

4 Grill for 2 minutes per side, or until no pink remains. Serve immediately.

Thumbs-up for gluten-free meal plans!

Exchanges
2 Very Lean Meat
1 Fat

Calories 117	
Calories from Fat . . . 35	
Total Fat . . . . 4 g	
Saturated Fat . . . . . . 0.7 g	
Cholesterol . . . . 49 mg	
Sodium . . . . 207 mg	
Total Carbohydrate . . . . 1 g	
Dietary Fiber . . . . 0 g	
Sugars . . . . 0 g	
Protein . . . . 18 g	

"Rain or shine, you'll enjoy these tangy skewers, 'cause they can also be cooked on an indoor grill or, if you prefer, under the broiler for about 2 minutes per side. Serve them by themselves or lay them across a bed of field greens for a light lunch or dinner. Either way, they're a real time-saver when you're in a pinch."

Nicole's Chicken Fingers

Serving Size: 2 pieces; Total Servings: 6

Nonstick cooking spray*

2/3 cup Fiber One cereal*

1 cup bran cereal*

1/4 cup chopped pecans

1 tablespoon sesame seeds

1/4 teaspoon salt

1/4 teaspoon ground red pepper*

2 egg whites

1 pound boneless, skinless chicken breast, cut into 12 strips

*To make this a gluten-free recipe, use gluten-free cereals and/or crispy coating mix, seasoning with no added starch from a gluten-containing source, and nonstick cooking spray with no flour added.

1 Preheat the oven to 350°F. Coat a baking sheet with nonstick cooking spray.

2 In a resealable plastic storage bag, combine the cereals, pecans, sesame seeds, salt, and red pepper. Crush into medium-fine crumbs then pour into a shallow dish. Place the egg whites in another shallow dish.

3 Dip each chicken strip into the egg whites then into the crumb mixture, coating completely. Place on the baking sheet and coat lightly with nonstick cooking spray.

4 Bake the chicken for 15 to 18 minutes, or until no pink remains. Serve immediately.

Exchanges
1 Starch
2 Lean Meat

Calories 190
   Calories from Fat . . . 61
Total Fat . . . . 7 g
   Saturated Fat . . . . . . 1.0 g
Cholesterol . . . . 44 mg
Sodium . . . . 243 mg
Total Carbohydrate . . . 18 g
   Dietary Fiber . . . . 8 g
   Sugars . . . . 4 g
Protein . . . . 20 g

"A real Southern tradition like fried chicken can be hard to give up when you switch to a diabetes meal plan. By coating boneless, skinless chicken with flavorful seasonings and baking it in the oven, we leave out the excess fat and calories and end up with a new, healthier way of enjoying an old favorite!"

Asian Meatballs

Serving Size: 3 meatballs; Total Servings: 8

1 pound extra-lean ground turkey breast

1 small onion, finely chopped

1/2 medium-sized green bell pepper, finely chopped

1/4 cup Panko bread crumbs*

2 egg whites

1/2 teaspoon garlic powder*

1/4 teaspoon ground red pepper*

1/2 teaspoon salt

1/4 teaspoon black pepper

1 tablespoon canola oil

1/4 cup plum sauce*

1 In a medium bowl, combine the turkey, onion, bell pepper, bread crumbs, egg whites, garlic powder, ground red pepper, salt, and black pepper. Shape into 24 one-inch meatballs.

2 In a large skillet, heat the oil over medium heat. Add the meatballs, cover, and cook for 8 to 10 minutes, or until no pink remains, turning occasionally to brown on all sides.

3 In a large bowl, combine the meatballs and the plum sauce, tossing to coat completely. Serve immediately.

*To make this a gluten-free recipe, use gluten-free plum sauce and bread crumb product and seasonings with no added starch from a gluten-containing source.

Exchanges

1/2 Carbohydrate
2 Very Lean Meat

Calories 104
    Calories from Fat . . . 19
Total Fat . . . . 2 g
    Saturated Fat . . . . . . 0.2 g
Cholesterol . . . . 31 mg
Sodium . . . . 289 mg
Total Carbohydrate . . . . 8 g
    Dietary Fiber . . . . 0 g
    Sugars . . . . 5 g
Protein . . . . 13 g

"One of my favorite things about this recipe is that we can use extra-lean ground turkey, which is normally 85 to 99% fat-free! And since protein is an important part of a diabetes meal plan, incorporating healthier choices such as lean ground turkey or beef is an easy option."

Tropical Shrimp

Serving Size: 4 shrimp; Total Servings: 7

1 tablespoon peanut oil

3 scallions, thinly sliced

2 teaspoons curry powder*

1/2 teaspoon ground ginger*

1/2 teaspoon chili powder*

1/4 teaspoon salt

1/4 teaspoon black pepper

3/4 cup plus 1 tablespoon light coconut milk

1 tablespoon fresh lime juice

1 teaspoon sugar

1 pound large shrimp, peeled and deveined, with tails left on (about 28)

1 In a large skillet, heat the oil over medium heat. Add the scallions and sauté for 1 minute. Add the curry powder, ginger, chili powder, salt, and pepper. Stir until the scallions are well coated with the seasonings.

2 Add the coconut milk, lime juice, and sugar; bring to a boil. Reduce the heat to low and simmer until the sauce reduces and thickens, about 5 minutes.

3 Add the shrimp and sauté for about 3 minutes, stirring constantly, until they turn pink. Serve immediately.

*To make this a gluten-free recipe, use seasonings with no added starch from a gluten-containing source.

Exchanges
1 Very Lean Meat
1 Fat

Calories	79
Calories from Fat . . .	35
Total Fat	4 g
Saturated Fat	1.4 g
Cholesterol	75 mg
Sodium	183 mg
Total Carbohydrate	3 g
Dietary Fiber	0 g
Sugars	1 g
Protein	8 g

"One of my personal favorites, this dish takes me back to a sunny beach in the Caribbean! The sweet and savory flavor combination is a huge hit on weeknights and whenever I entertain. It always has my friends and family raving. And the best part? It takes only minutes to dish up, so it always fits my busy schedule."

Out-of-the-Ordinary Rumaki

Serving Size: 2 wraps; Total Servings: 13

1/3 cup ketchup

2 tablespoons white vinegar

1 tablespoon light brown sugar

1/4 teaspoon hot pepper sauce

6 ounces turkey bacon (about 13 strips), each strip cut in half

1 pound sea scallops, rinsed and patted dry (about 26)

1 In a large bowl, combine the ketchup, vinegar, brown sugar, and hot pepper sauce; stir until smooth.

2 Roll a piece of bacon around each scallop and secure each with a wooden toothpick. Place in the ketchup mixture and toss gently to coat. Cover and chill for 20 minutes.

3 Preheat the broiler. Line a rimmed baking sheet with aluminum foil.

4 Place the bacon-wrapped scallops on the baking sheet, discarding the remaining marinade. Broil for 4 to 5 minutes per side, or until the scallops are cooked through.

Exchanges
1 Very Lean Meat
1/2 Fat

Calories 68
Calories from Fat . . . 22
Total Fat . . . . 2 g
Saturated Fat . . . . . . 0.7 g
Cholesterol . . . . 21 mg
Sodium . . . . 315 mg
Total Carbohydrate . . . . 3 g
Dietary Fiber . . . . 0 g
Sugars . . . . 2 g
Protein . . . . 8 g

"Rumaki is traditionally made with chicken livers, water chestnuts, and pork bacon. This is a much lighter version that you just may like even better, thanks to the terrific sauce. You might even want to make it your own by wrapping shrimp, chunks of tender chicken breast, or a mild, firm fish like cod, grouper, sea bass, or mahimahi instead of scallops."

Smoked Salmon Rounds

Serving Size: 3 rounds; Total Servings: 10

3 ounces light cream cheese, softened

1 scallion, thinly sliced

30 Melba toast rounds (about 2/3 of a 5-1/4 ounce box)*

1 package (3 ounces) smoked salmon, cut into 30 pieces

1 tablespoon minced red onion

1 In a small bowl, combine the cream cheese and scallion; mix well.

2 Spread the cream cheese mixture evenly over the Melba toast rounds. Place 1 piece of smoked salmon on top of each and sprinkle with minced onion.

*To make this a gluten-free recipe, use gluten-free rice crackers instead of Melba toast rounds.

Exchanges
1/2 Starch
1/2 Fat

Calories 70
　Calories from Fat . . . 22
Total Fat . . . . 2 g
　Saturated Fat . . . . . . 1.3 g
Cholesterol . . . . 8 mg
Sodium . . . . 185 mg
Total Carbohydrate . . . . 8 g
　Dietary Fiber . . . . 1 g
　Sugars . . . . 1 g
Protein . . . . 4 g

Finishing Touch

Make these extra special by garnishing each round with a small sprig of fresh dill, in addition to or instead of the minced red onion. Now that's what I like to call the "wow" factor!

Buffalo Catfish Strips

Serving Size: 2 strips; Total Servings: 9

Nonstick cooking spray

2 tablespoons all-purpose flour

1 teaspoon garlic powder

1 teaspoon paprika

1 teaspoon onion powder

1/2 teaspoon salt

1/8 teaspoon ground red pepper

1/3 cup buffalo wing sauce

1-1/2 cups coarsely crushed cornflakes

1 pound catfish fillets, cut into 18 strips

1 Preheat the oven to 400°F. Coat a baking sheet with nonstick cooking spray.

2 In a shallow dish, combine the flour, garlic powder, paprika, onion powder, salt, and red pepper; mix well.

3 Place the wing sauce in a second shallow dish and the crushed cornflakes in a third shallow dish.

4 Coat the fish strips in the flour mixture, dip in the wing sauce then roll in the crushed cornflakes, coating completely. Place the fish strips on the baking sheet and lightly coat the tops with nonstick cooking spray.

5 Bake for 8 to 10 minutes, or until the fish flakes easily with a fork. Serve immediately.

Exchanges
1/2 Starch
1 Lean Meat

Calories 107
Calories from Fat . . . 30
Total Fat . . . . 3 g
Saturated Fat . . . . . . 1.1 g
Cholesterol . . . . 27 mg
Sodium . . . . 425 mg
Total Carbohydrate . . . . 8 g
Dietary Fiber . . . . 0 g
Sugars . . . . 1 g
Protein . . . . 10 g

Preparation Tip

Go ahead and make these as mild or hot as you'd like. Just choose the amount of paprika and ground red pepper and the intensity of the wing sauce that you want. No matter which way you serve 'em, your gang will be hooked!

Salads & Dressings

Tomato and Artichoke Salad

Serving Size: 1 cup; Total Servings: 6

6 plum tomatoes, cut into 1-inch chunks (about 1-1/2 pounds)

1 can (14 ounces) artichoke hearts, drained and quartered

1/2 sweet onion, cut into 1-inch chunks

1/3 cup light balsamic dressing*

1/4 cup crumbled real blue cheese

1 In a large bowl, toss all the ingredients until well combined. Serve immediately, or cover and chill until ready to serve.

*To make this a gluten-free recipe, use dressing with no added starch from a gluten-containing source.

Exchanges
2 Vegetable
1/2 Fat

Calories 74
   Calories from Fat . . . 32
Total Fat . . . . 4 g
   Saturated Fat . . . . . . 1.1 g
Cholesterol . . . . 4 mg
Sodium . . . . 391 mg
Total Carbohydrate . . . . 9 g
   Dietary Fiber . . . . 2 g
   Sugars . . . . 4 g
Protein . . . . 3 g

"There may be only five ingredients in this unusual salad, but it's not short on taste! Between the robust balsamic dressing and the tangy blue cheese (which is one of my all-time favorites for adding tons of flavor in small amounts), it's a winning combination."

Marinated Steak Salad

Serving Size: 2 cups; Total Servings: 6

2 tablespoons olive oil

Juice of 1 lime

1 small onion, minced

1 tablespoon crushed red pepper*

1/4 teaspoon salt

1 pound beef flank steak

Nonstick cooking spray*

1 head romaine lettuce, cut into bite-sized pieces

6 plum tomatoes, sliced into wedges

2 tablespoons sliced olives

2 tablespoons crumbled reduced-fat real feta cheese

See photo, opposite.

1 In a large resealable plastic bag, combine the oil, lime juice, onion, crushed red pepper, and salt; mix well. Add the steak then seal; turn to coat. Marinate in the refrigerator for at least 4 hours, turning occasionally.

2 Drain the steak, discarding the marinade.

3 Coat a medium skillet with non-stick cooking spray. Heat the skillet over high heat, add the steak, and cook for 4 to 5 minutes per side for medium-rare or to desired doneness. Slice the steak thinly across the grain.

4 Place the lettuce on a platter; arrange the steak slices and tomato wedges over it. Sprinkle with olives and cheese, and serve.

*To make this a gluten-free recipe, use seasonings with no added starch from a gluten-containing source and nonstick cooking spray with no flour added.

Exchanges
1 Vegetable
2 Lean Meat
1/2 Fat

Calories 161
  Calories from Fat . . . 66
Total Fat . . . . 7 g
  Saturated Fat . . . . . . 2.4 g
Cholesterol . . . . 27 mg
Sodium . . . . 162 mg
Total Carbohydrate . . . . 7 g
  Dietary Fiber . . . . 3 g
  Sugars . . . . 4 g
Protein . . . . 17 g

Preparation Tip

To save time, marinate the steak the night before. Then, when you're ready, cook the meat and prepare the salad. Squeeze it with a fresh lime or top with low-fat dressing.

Marinated Steak Salad

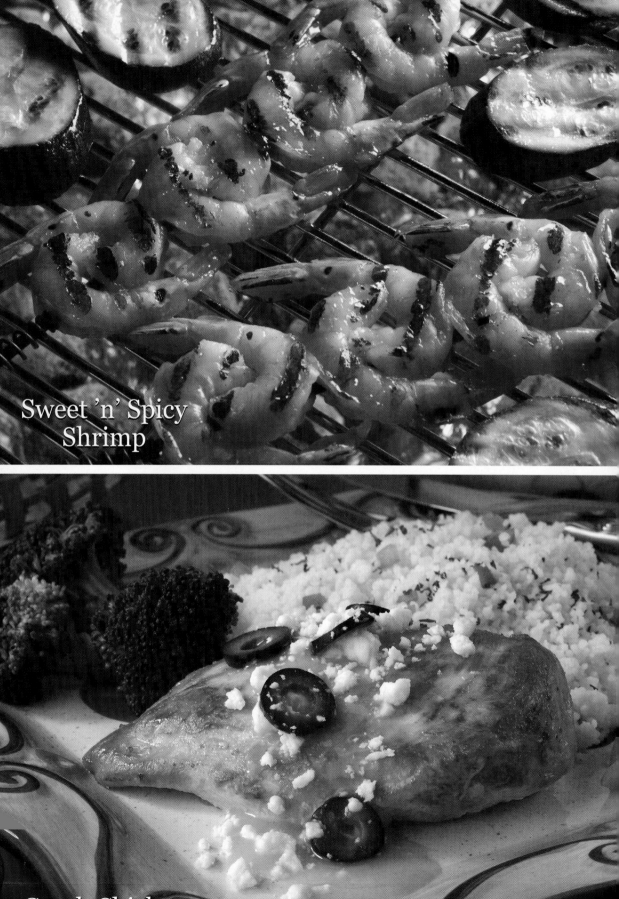

Sweet 'n' Spicy
Shrimp

Greek Chicken

Cheesy Spinach Quiche

Kung Pao Beef

Confetti Cottage Cheese

Serving Size: 3/4 cup; Total Servings: 4

1 container (16 ounces) low-fat cottage cheese

6 radishes, chopped

2 scallions, thinly sliced

1/2 medium cucumber, seeded and chopped

1 tablespoon chopped fresh dill weed

1/4 teaspoon salt

1/4 teaspoon black pepper

4 romaine lettuce leaves

1 In a medium bowl, combine all the ingredients except the lettuce; mix well.

2 Place lettuce leaves on individual serving plates and top each with equal amounts of cottage cheese mixture. Serve immediately.

Thumbs-up for gluten-free meal plans!

Exchanges

1 Vegetable
2 Very Lean Meat

Calories 93
    Calories from Fat . . . 12
Total Fat . . . . 1 g
    Saturated Fat . . . . . . 0.8 g
Cholesterol . . . . 5 mg
Sodium . . . . 612 mg
Total Carbohydrate . . . . 6 g
    Dietary Fiber . . . . 1 g
    Sugars . . . . 4 g
Protein . . . . 15 g

"Did you know that cottage cheese is loaded with protein and calcium? It's a 'good for you' food that's part of many different meal plans. I like to enjoy it as part of a salad, as in this recipe, or pair it with berries and other fresh fruit for a light snack. Mr. Food says it's best to use large-curd cottage cheese here, because it stands up better when mixed with the fresh veggies . . . and I always take Mr. Food's recipe suggestions!"

"Beet"-the-Clock Spinach Salad

Serving Size: 1/8 recipe; Total Servings: 8

1/3 cup canola oil

3 tablespoons apple cider vinegar

1 tablespoon honey

1 teaspoon onion powder*

1 teaspoon garlic powder*

1/2 teaspoon salt

1/2 teaspoon black pepper

1 package (10 ounces) fresh spinach

1 can (8-1/4 ounces) julienne beets, drained

1/4 cup imitation bacon bits*

1 In a medium saucepan, bring the oil, vinegar, honey, onion powder, garlic powder, salt, and black pepper to a boil over medium heat.

2 In a large bowl, combine the spinach, drained beets, and bacon bits. Pour the hot dressing over the spinach mixture; toss to coat well. Serve immediately.

---

*To make this a gluten-free recipe, use seasonings with no added starch from a gluten-containing source and gluten-free imitation bacon bits.

Exchanges
1 Vegetable
2 Fat

Calories 118
Calories from Fat . . . 89
Total Fat . . . . 10 g
Saturated Fat . . . . . . 0.8 g
Cholesterol . . . . 0 mg
Sodium . . . . 253 mg
Total Carbohydrate . . . . 6 g
Dietary Fiber . . . . 1 g
Sugars . . . . 4 g
Protein . . . . 2 g

Preparation Tip

Be sure to take extra care when working with beets (canned or fresh) because of their tendency to stain anything from hands to clothing.

Asparagus and Tomato Salad

Serving Size: 1 cup; Total Servings: 8

2 packages (10 ounces each) frozen asparagus spears, thawed and cut in half (see Option)

4 large plum tomatoes, cut into 1-inch chunks (1 pound)

1/2 red onion, cut into strips

2 tablespoons extra virgin olive oil

1 tablespoon balsamic vinegar

1/4 cup chopped fresh basil

3/4 teaspoon salt

1 In a large bowl, combine the asparagus, tomatoes, and onion; toss gently.

2 In a small bowl, whisk together the remaining ingredients. Pour over the asparagus mixture and toss until coated.

3 Cover and chill for at least 1 hour before serving.

Thumbs-up for gluten-free meal plans!

Option

If you'd prefer to use fresh asparagus, simply blanch them in a large pot of boiling water for 2 minutes then cool and cut.

Exchanges

1 Vegetable
1 Fat

Calories	64
Calories from Fat	34
Total Fat	4 g
Saturated Fat	0.5 g
Cholesterol	0 mg
Sodium	224 mg
Total Carbohydrate	7 g
Dietary Fiber	2 g
Sugars	3 g
Protein	3 g

"Including tomatoes (probably my favorite food) in any meal plan is a smart choice because they're packed with lycopene—a natural compound that gives fruits and veggies their bright colors and supports the immune system. Tomatoes also contain antioxidants, which may provide protection from certain types of cancers. With all that tomatoes have to offer, enjoy their benefits all year long!"

Chinese Chicken Salad

Serving Size: 1-2/3 cups; Total Servings: 8

1 tablespoon peanut oil

4 garlic cloves, minced

1/3 cup dry-roasted, unsalted peanuts

2 tablespoons light soy sauce*

2 tablespoons white vinegar

3 tablespoons sugar

3-1/2 tablespoons canola oil

1 head Napa or Chinese cabbage, washed and cut into bite-sized pieces

2 cups cooked chunked boneless, skinless chicken breast (12 ounces) (see Tips)

1 small carrot, shredded

1 In a medium saucepan, heat the peanut oil over medium heat. Add the garlic and peanuts and sauté for 3 to 5 minutes, until the garlic is lightly toasted.

2 Reduce the heat to medium-low and add the soy sauce, vinegar, sugar, and canola oil. Cook for 2 minutes, until heated through.

3 In a large bowl, combine the cabbage, chicken, and carrot. Pour the warm dressing over the cabbage mixture; toss until well coated. Serve immediately.

*To make this a gluten-free recipe, use gluten-free soy sauce or pure tamari.

Exchanges
1/2 Carbohydrate
1 Vegetable
2 Lean Meat
1 Fat

Calories 211	
Calories from Fat . . 111	
Total Fat . . . . 2 g	
Saturated Fat . . . . . . 1.6 g	
Cholesterol . . . . 36 mg	
Sodium . . . . 187 mg	
Total Carbohydrate . . . 10 g	
Dietary Fiber . . . . 2 g	
Sugars . . . . 7 g	
Protein . . . . 16 g	

Serving Tips

You can use leftover chicken or store-bought, precooked chicken in this main-dish salad. If you have the time, simply trim any visible fat from 1 pound boneless, skinless chicken breast and place the chicken in a saucepan. Add just enough water to cover and bring to a boil over medium-high heat. Reduce heat to medium-low and simmer for 10 to 15 minutes, or until no pink remains in the chicken. Remove the chicken from the water and let cool. Cut into bite-sized chunks, cover, and chill until ready to use. It's that easy!

Southwestern Chicken Salad

Serving Size: 1 cup; Total Servings: 4

6 plum tomatoes, chopped

2 cups cooked, chunked boneless, skinless chicken breast (12 ounces) (See Tips, page 40)

1/2 red onion, chopped

2 jalapeño peppers, seeded and minced

2 garlic cloves, minced

3 tablespoons fresh lime juice

2 tablespoons finely chopped fresh cilantro

3/4 teaspoon salt

1/4 teaspoon black pepper

1 In a large bowl, combine all the ingredients; mix well. Cover and chill for at least 1 hour before serving.

Thumbs-up for gluten-free meal plans!

Exchanges

2 Vegetable
3 Very Lean Meat
1/2 Fat

Calories 189	
Calories from Fat . . . 31	
Total Fat . . . . 3 g	
Saturated Fat . . . . . . 0.9 g	
Cholesterol . . . . 72 mg	
Sodium . . . . 511 mg	
Total Carbohydrate . . . 11 g	
Dietary Fiber . . . . 3 g	
Sugars . . . . 7 g	
Protein . . . . 28 g	

"Turn your next week-night dinner into a colorful fiesta with this throw-together chicken salad. Serve each portion on a romaine lettuce leaf or with a low-fat tortilla. Even without mayonnaise or salad dressing, this chicken salad is bound to have your family saying, 'Ay qué bueno!' That's Spanish for 'OOH IT'S SO GOOD!!'"

Grilled Summer Salad

Serving Size: 1-1/2 cups; Total Servings: 8

1 pound boneless, skinless chicken breast

1 pound fresh asparagus, trimmed

2 packages (5 ounces each) mixed baby greens

1/2 pint grape tomatoes, halved

1/2 cup frozen corn, thawed

1/2 cup crumbled real feta cheese

1/3 cup sliced almonds, toasted

1/3 cup chopped dates*

1/2 cup reduced-fat raspberry vinaigrette

1 Preheat the grill to medium.

2 Grill the chicken and asparagus for 5 to 6 minutes per side, or until the chicken is no longer pink and the asparagus is tender. Remove from the grill; slice into bite-sized pieces.

3 In a large salad bowl, toss together the remaining ingredients. Top with the chicken and asparagus, drizzle with the dressing, and serve.

*To make this a gluten-free recipe, use dates that have not been dusted with wheat flour to prevent sticking.

Exchanges
1 Carbohydrate
2 Lean Meat
1/2 Fat

Calories 196
  Calories from Fat . . . 76
Total Fat . . . . 8 g
  Saturated Fat . . . . . . 2.1 g
Cholesterol . . . . 42 mg
Sodium . . . . 279 mg
Total Carbohydrate . . . 15 g
  Dietary Fiber . . . . 3 g
  Sugars . . . . 10 g
Protein . . . . 16 g

"Tired of the same ho-hum potato salad that seems to be the standard side dish served at every picnic and backyard barbecue? This is one of my favorite recipes for jazzing things up while keeping it all oh-so-sweet and simple!"

Minty Chicken Salad

Serving Size: 1-1/2 cups; Total Servings: 8

2 cups cooked, chunked chicken breast

1/2 yellow bell pepper, chopped

1/2 red bell pepper, chopped

1/2 cup cubed cucumber

1/2 cup (2 ounces) crumbled reduced-fat real feta cheese

1/4 cup chopped fresh mint

2 tablespoons fresh lemon juice

1-1/2 teaspoons olive oil

1 teaspoon dried oregano*

1/4 teaspoon salt

1/4 teaspoon black pepper

1 package (10 ounces) mixed lettuce greens

1 In a large bowl, combine all the ingredients except the mixed lettuce greens; toss until well combined.

2 Place the mixed greens on a platter and top with the chicken mixture. Serve immediately, or cover and chill until ready to serve.

*To make this a gluten-free recipe, use seasonings with no added starch from a gluten-containing source.

Exchanges
1 Vegetable
2 Very Lean Meat
1/2 Fat

Calories 109
  Calories from Fat . . . 33
Total Fat . . . . 4 g
  Saturated Fat . . . . . . 1.3 g
Cholesterol . . . . 39 mg
Sodium . . . . 227 mg
Total Carbohydrate . . . . 3 g
  Dietary Fiber . . . . 1 g
  Sugars . . . . 2 g
Protein . . . . 16 g

"Fresh mint is a terrific way to perk up practically any dish! It's available throughout the year, so wake up your next meal and surprise the gang with the fresh taste of mint in this main-dish salad!"

Speedy Fajita Salad

Serving Size: 1-1/2 cups; Total Servings: 6

1 tablespoon canola oil

2 large onions, cut into
8 wedges each

2 large bell peppers (1 yellow
and 1 green), cut into
1/2-inch strips

1 pound boneless, skinless
chicken breast, cut into
1/2-inch strips

2 tablespoons dry fajita
seasoning

1/2 medium head iceberg lettuce,
shredded (about 4 cups)

1/2 cup salsa

1 In a large skillet, heat the oil over medium-high heat. Add the onions and peppers and sauté for 3 to 5 minutes, or until the onions are tender, stirring occasionally.

2 In a small bowl, combine the chicken and fajita seasoning; toss until the chicken is thoroughly coated. Add to the skillet and cook for 5 to 6 minutes, or until no pink remains in the chicken and the onions are browned, stirring frequently.

3 Place the shredded lettuce on a serving platter, top with the chicken mixture, and drizzle with salsa. Serve immediately.

Exchanges
3 Vegetable
2 Very Lean Meat
1/2 Fat

Calories 167
Calories from Fat . . . 39
Total Fat . . . . 4 g
Saturated Fat . . . . . . 0.7 g
Cholesterol . . . . 44 mg
Sodium . . . . 375 mg
Total Carbohydrate . . . 15 g
Dietary Fiber . . . . 3 g
Sugars . . . . 7 g
Protein . . . . 18 g

"There's nothing like the smell and the sizzle of a hot plate of fajitas being served up. And now we can enjoy that scrumptious experience with a salad! Add sizzle to your menu with this family favorite, maybe even substituting a tender cut of beef for the chicken or topping each serving with a dollop of low-fat sour cream or a slice of avocado. It's all up to you!"

Perfectly Peachy Waldorf Salad

Serving Size: 1 cup; Total Servings: 5

2 cups cooked, chunked boneless, skinless chicken breast (12 ounces) (see Tips, page 40)

2 medium peaches, pitted and chopped (see below)

1/3 cup walnuts, coarsely chopped and toasted

1 rib celery, diced

1/2 red bell pepper, diced

1/3 cup light mayonnaise

1 tablespoon honey

1/2 teaspoon salt

1/4 teaspoon black pepper

5 whole-grain rolls (2 ounces each)

1 In a large bowl, combine the chicken, peaches, walnuts, celery, and bell pepper.

2 In a small bowl, combine the mayonnaise, honey, salt, and black pepper; mix well.

3 Pour the mayonnaise mixture over the chicken mixture; toss gently. Cover and chill for at least 2 hours, or until ready to serve with the rolls.

Exchanges
1-1/2 Starch
1 Fruit
3 Very Lean Meat
2-1/2 Fat

Calories 381	
Calories from Fat . . 134	
Total Fat . . . . 15 g	
Saturated Fat . . . . . . 2.4 g	
Cholesterol . . . . 63 mg	
Sodium . . . . 660 mg	
Total Carbohydrate . . . 36 g	
Dietary Fiber . . . . 3 g	
Sugars . . . . 13 g	
Protein . . . . 26 g	

"Since we all usually have these everyday ingredients on hand, Waldorf salad can't get much easier! Of course, I like to switch things around each time by using different fruit, so try pears, mandarin oranges, or whatever fresh fruit you like, as long as the numbers still work for you. This is a fast and simple meal that looks so gourmet-fancy!"

Tabbouleh Salad

Serving Size: 3/4 cup; Total Servings: 7

1 cup bulgur wheat*

2 cups hot water

1 tablespoon olive oil

1/3 cup fresh lemon juice

1 teaspoon minced garlic

2 teaspoons dried mint

1 teaspoon salt

1/4 teaspoon black pepper

1 medium tomato, finely chopped

1/2 small cucumber, finely chopped

6 scallions, thinly sliced

2 cups coarsely chopped fresh parsley (see Note)

1 In a large bowl, combine the bulgur wheat and water; allow to stand for 20 to 30 minutes, or until the water is completely absorbed.

2 Add the oil, lemon juice, garlic, mint, salt, and pepper; mix until thoroughly combined. Add the remaining ingredients and toss until blended.

3 Cover and chill for at least 1 hour before serving.

---

*To make this a gluten-free recipe, use quinoa granules instead of bulgur wheat.

Exchanges
1 Starch
1 Vegetable
1/2 Fat

Calories 117
  Calories from Fat . . . 22
Total Fat . . . . 2 g
  Saturated Fat . . . . . . 0.3 g
Cholesterol . . . . 0 mg
Sodium . . . . 353 mg
Total Carbohydrate . . . 22 g
  Dietary Fiber . . . . 6 g
  Sugars . . . . 2 g
Protein . . . . 4 g

"If you're always on the go, like I am, this zippy Mediterranean salad will be perfect for you! It makes a quick snack, a simple lunch, and even a great go-along for whatever you're serving for dinner. And don't get scared by the amount of chopped parsley it calls for. An easy way to chop it without really chopping is to just snip the parsley leaves off the stems in small pieces with a pair of handy kitchen shears."

Tuna Antipasto

Serving Size: 1-1/2 cups; Total Servings: 6

1 large can (12 ounces) water-packed solid white tuna, drained

1/2 medium head iceberg lettuce, coarsely chopped (about 4 cups)

1 medium tomato, cut into 1-inch chunks

1 medium cucumber, peeled and cut into 1-inch chunks

1 small red onion, cut into 1-inch chunks

1 jar (12 ounces) jardinière marinated vegetables, rinsed and drained

1/2 cup light Italian dressing

1 Flake the tuna into a large bowl. Add the remaining ingredients; toss to mix. Serve immediately.

Option

For a more robust flavor, substitute 1/2 cup of my Sun-Dried Tomato Vinaigrette (page 53) for the Italian dressing.

Exchanges

1 Vegetable
2 Very Lean Meat

Calories 100
  Calories from Fat . . . 15
Total Fat . . . . 2 g
  Saturated Fat . . . . . . 0.3 g
Cholesterol . . . . 15 mg
Sodium . . . . 734 mg
Total Carbohydrate . . . . 6 g
  Dietary Fiber . . . . 2 g
  Sugars . . . . 4 g
Protein . . . . 14 g

California Tuna Salad

1 large can (12 ounces) water-packed solid white tuna, drained

1 can (15 ounces) cannellini beans (white kidney beans), rinsed and drained

1 can (15 ounces) red kidney beans, rinsed and drained

1/2 cup hot salsa

6 scallions, thinly sliced

1 tablespoon lemon juice

1 teaspoon minced garlic

1 teaspoon dried basil*

1/2 teaspoon ground cumin*

1 Flake the tuna into a large bowl. Add the remaining ingredients; toss to mix.

2 Cover and chill for at least 1 hour, or until ready to serve.

*To make this a gluten-free recipe, use seasonings with no added starch from a gluten-containing source.

Exchanges
2 Starch
2 Very Lean Meat

Calories 233
  Calories from Fat . . . 11
Total Fat . . . . 1 g
  Saturated Fat . . . . . . 0.2 g
Cholesterol . . . . 18 mg
Sodium . . . . 520 mg
Total Carbohydrate . . . 30 g
  Dietary Fiber . . . . 8 g
  Sugars . . . . 3 g
Protein . . . . 26 g

"Want to add a little extra flair? Serve this West Coast refresher on a bed of romaine or colorful Salad Savoy. This one will definitely reel in the applause!"

Cilantro Shrimp Salad

Serving Size: 3/4 cup; Total Servings: 8

- 1/2 pound cooked large salad shrimp, peeled and deveined
- 1 can (15 ounces) black beans, drained and rinsed
- 1 medium-sized cucumber, chopped
- 1 cup frozen corn, thawed
- 1/2 medium-sized red bell pepper, chopped
- 1/3 cup chopped fresh cilantro
- 1/2 cup canola oil
- Juice of 1 lime (3 tablespoons)
- 1 tablespoon white vinegar
- 1 teaspoon sugar
- 1/2 teaspoon crushed red pepper*
- 1/4 teaspoon salt
- 1/4 teaspoon black pepper

1 In a large bowl, combine the shrimp, black beans, cucumber, corn, bell pepper, and cilantro; mix well and set aside.

2 In a medium bowl, combine the remaining ingredients; mix well and pour over the shrimp mixture, tossing until well coated. Cover and chill for at least 1 hour before serving.

---

*To make this a gluten-free recipe, use seasonings with no added starch from a gluten-containing source.

Exchanges
1 Starch
1 Very Lean Meat
2-1/2 Fat

Calories	212
Calories from Fat . .	131
Total Fat	15 g
Saturated Fat	1.1 g
Cholesterol	45 mg
Sodium	165 mg
Total Carbohydrate . . .	13 g
Dietary Fiber	3 g
Sugars	2 g
Protein	8 g

Did You Know . . .

that according to folklore, cilantro was hailed by Greek and Roman doctors for its medicinal powers? It's also believed to have been one of the earliest plantings in North America. Today, cilantro is popular in all types of cooking, from Mexican to Asian, Indian, and lots more.

Shrimp Salad Skewers

Serving Size: 2 skewers; Total Servings: 4

1/2 cup light ranch dressing*

2 teaspoons prepared horseradish

8 ten-inch wooden skewers

1 head iceberg lettuce, cut into 16 wedges

2 large tomatoes, each cut into 8 chunks

16 cooked shrimp, peeled and deveined, with tails left on (about 3/4 pound)

1 lemon, cut into 8 wedges

1 In a small bowl, combine the ranch dressing and horseradish; mix well, cover, and chill for 1 hour.

2 Thread each skewer, alternating ingredients, with 2 wedges of lettuce, 2 tomato chunks, and 2 shrimp; finish each with a lemon wedge.

3 Serve the kabobs drizzled with the dressing.

*To make this a gluten-free recipe, use dressing with no added starch from a gluten-containing source.

Exchanges

1/2 Carbohydrate
1 Vegetable
2 Very Lean Meat
1/2 Fat

Calories 157
  Calories from Fat . . . 45
Total Fat . . . . 5 g
  Saturated Fat . . . . . . 0.8 g
Cholesterol . . . . 108 mg
Sodium . . . . 490 mg
Total Carbohydrate . . . 14 g
  Dietary Fiber . . . . 3 g
  Sugars . . . . 5 g
Protein . . . . 13 g

"Forget the forks with this kid-friendly, hands-on treat! It's a sure way to beat the dinnertime rut, and it can even be prepared in advance . . . meaning it takes no time to get from preparation to the table. And if you combine the dressing in the morning or earlier in the day, that'll help get this low-carb pleaser on the table even quicker."

Red Wine Vinaigrette

Serving Size: 2 tablespoons; Total Servings: 10

7 tablespoons olive oil

1/2 cup red wine vinegar

2 garlic cloves, minced

1/4 cup finely chopped onion

1/4 cup finely chopped fresh parsley

1-1/2 teaspoons sugar

1/2 teaspoon salt

1/8 teaspoon black pepper

1 In a small bowl, combine all the ingredients and whisk until well combined.

2 Serve immediately or, for a mellower onion flavor, cover and chill for at least 2 hours before serving.

Thumbs-up for gluten-free meal plans!

Exchanges
2 Fat

Calories 91	
Calories from Fat . . . 85	
Total Fat . . . . 9 g	
Saturated Fat . . . . . . 1.3 g	
Cholesterol . . . . 0 mg	
Sodium . . . . 118 mg	
Total Carbohydrate . . . . 2 g	
Dietary Fiber . . . . 0 g	
Sugars . . . . 2 g	
Protein . . . . 0 g	

"Looking for a new addition to your dressing lineup? Look no further! Even on days when you're short on time, the convenience of bagged salads and ready-to-use chopped veggies means a quick and healthy salad isn't far away. Plus, my vinaigrette dressing is made up of everyday ingredients most of us have in the kitchen to begin with. It's as easy as 1-2-3!"

Creamy Balsamic Dressing

Serving Size: 2 tablespoons; Total Servings: 14

1 cup low-fat plain yogurt

1/4 cup light mayonnaise*

3 tablespoons Dijon mustard

2 tablespoons fresh lemon juice

1/3 cup balsamic vinegar

2 tablespoons honey

1 tablespoon dried parsley flakes*

1 In a small bowl, combine all the ingredients and blend with a spoon or whisk until smooth and creamy.

2 Serve, or cover and chill until ready to serve.

*To make this a gluten-free recipe, use gluten-free mayonnaise and dried parsley flakes with no added starch from a gluten-containing source.

Exchanges
1/2 Carbohydrate

Calories 42
   Calories from Fat . . . 16
Total Fat . . . . 2 g
   Saturated Fat . . . . . . 0.4 g
Cholesterol . . . . 3 mg
Sodium . . . . 127 mg
Total Carbohydrate . . . . 6 g
   Dietary Fiber . . . . 0 g
   Sugars . . . . 5 g
Protein . . . . 1 g

"Trust me—there's nothing like homemade dressing! And using low-fat plain yogurt instead of milk is a good-for-you way to create a creamy homemade dressing while still keeping the smooth flavor and texture of store-bought versions!"

Sun-Dried Tomato Vinaigrette

Serving Size: 2 tablespoons; Total Servings: 14

1/2 cup (2 ounces) sun-dried tomatoes, julienne-cut

1/2 cup olive oil

1/2 cup reduced-sodium chicken broth

1/3 cup balsamic vinegar

2 garlic cloves

1 teaspoon onion powder

1 teaspoon sugar

1/4 teaspoon salt

1/4 teaspoon black pepper

1 In a food processor or blender, combine all the ingredients and process until smooth, scraping down the sides as needed.

2 Serve, or cover and chill until ready to serve.

Exchanges
2 Fat

Calories	80
Calories from Fat	70
Total Fat	8 g
Saturated Fat	1.0 g
Cholesterol	0 mg
Sodium	60 mg
Total Carbohydrate	3 g
Dietary Fiber	0 g
Sugars	2 g
Protein	0 g

Preparation Tip

Jazz up your salad greens or other salads with this Italian-inspired dressing. It also makes a great marinade for roasting or grilling hearty veggies.

Japanese Ginger Dressing

Serving Size: 2 tablespoons; Total Servings: 14

1/2 cup chopped onion

1/2 cup peanut oil

1/4 cup white vinegar

1/4 cup water

2 tablespoons light soy sauce*

2 tablespoons lemon juice

2 tablespoons ketchup

2 teaspoons ground ginger*

2 teaspoons sugar

1/2 teaspoon salt

1/2 teaspoon black pepper

1 In a food processor or blender, combine all the ingredients and process until smooth, scraping down the sides as needed.

2 Serve, or cover and chill until ready to use.

*To make this a gluten-free recipe, use gluten-free soy sauce or pure tamari and seasonings with no added starch from a gluten-containing source.

Exchanges
2 Fat

Calories 79
Calories from Fat . . . 70
Total Fat . . . . 8 g
Saturated Fat . . . . . . 1.3 g
Cholesterol . . . . 0 mg
Sodium . . . . 191 mg
Total Carbohydrate . . . . 3 g
Dietary Fiber . . . . 0 g
Sugars . . . . 2 g
Protein . . . . 0 g

"If you've ever been to a traditional Japanese restaurant or sushi bar, you know how sweet and tangy this dressing usually is—and my homemade version will have everybody grabbing their chopsticks! Make a quick Japanese salad by tossing fresh iceberg or romaine lettuce leaves in a bowl with sliced tomato and cucumber then topping it with this ginger dressing."

Soups

Creamy Zucchini Soup

Serving Size: 1 cup; Total Servings: 8

Nonstick cooking spray

1 large onion, chopped

1/2 red bell pepper, minced

3 garlic cloves, minced

1-1/2 pounds zucchini, chopped into 1/2-inch cubes

2 cans (14 ounces each) reduced-sodium chicken broth

2 tablespoons chopped fresh dill weed

1/2 teaspoon salt

1/4 teaspoon black pepper

1 cup low-fat milk

3 tablespoons cornstarch

1 Coat a soup pot with nonstick cooking spray and heat over medium-high heat.

2 Add the onion, bell pepper, and garlic, and sauté for 4 to 5 minutes, or until tender, stirring frequently.

3 Add the zucchini, chicken broth, dill weed, salt, and black pepper; bring to a boil. Reduce the heat to low, cover, and simmer for 25 to 30 minutes, or until the zucchini is tender.

4 In a small bowl, whisk together the milk and cornstarch until smooth; add to the soup mixture, stirring until thickened. Ladle into bowls and serve.

Exchanges
1 Carbohydrate

Calories	60
Calories from Fat	4
Total Fat	0 g
Saturated Fat	0.2 g
Cholesterol	2 mg
Sodium	412 mg
Total Carbohydrate	11 g
Dietary Fiber	2 g
Sugars	5 g
Protein	4 g

"By using a combination of cornstarch and low-fat milk, instead of heavy cream, we've reduced the fat and calories from the traditional version of this soup while keeping its rich 'n' creamy texture."

Tomato Florentine Soup

Serving Size: 1 cup; Total Servings: 7

1 teaspoon olive oil

1 large onion, chopped

3 garlic cloves, minced

3 large tomatoes, diced (about 2 pounds)

2 teaspoons Italian seasoning

2 cans (14 ounces each) reduced-sodium chicken broth

1 package (10 ounces) fresh spinach, trimmed

1/2 teaspoon black pepper

2 tablespoons grated Parmesan cheese (optional)

1 In a soup pot, heat the oil over medium heat. Add the onion and garlic and sauté for 5 minutes, or until the onion is browned, stirring occasionally.

2 Add the tomatoes and Italian seasoning and cook for 10 minutes, or until the tomatoes soften, stirring occasionally.

3 Add the chicken broth, spinach, and pepper; bring to a boil. Reduce the heat to low, cover, and simmer for 2 to 3 minutes, or until the spinach is wilted.

4 Ladle soup into bowls, sprinkle with Parmesan cheese, if desired, and serve.

Exchanges
2 Vegetable

Calories 61
   Calories from Fat . . . 10
Total Fat . . . . 1 g
   Saturated Fat . . . . . . 0.2 g
Cholesterol . . . . 0 mg
Sodium . . . . 315 mg
Total Carbohydrate . . . 11 g
   Dietary Fiber . . . . 3 g
   Sugars . . . . 5 g
Protein . . . . 4 g

"Some nights, a quick bowl of warm and soothing soup is all that can satisfy our tummies (and our schedules). This homestyle favorite is an easy way to keep healthy green veggies, like spinach, in your meal plan."

Split Pea Soup

Serving Size: 1 cup; Total Servings: 5

1 bag (14 ounces) dried split peas, rinsed and cleaned according to package directions

7 cups water

2 beef bouillon cubes

1 medium onion, finely chopped

1 cup grated carrots (2 to 3 carrots)

1/2 teaspoon black pepper

1 In a soup pot, combine all the ingredients; mix well. Bring to a boil over medium-high heat.

2 Reduce the heat to medium-low and simmer for 1 hour, or until the peas are soft and thoroughly cooked.

Exchanges

3 Starch
1 Very Lean Meat

Calories	262
Calories from Fat	8
Total Fat	1 g
Saturated Fat	0.1 g
Cholesterol	0 mg
Sodium	393 mg
Total Carbohydrate . . .	48 g
Dietary Fiber	18 g
Sugars	8 g
Protein	17 g

"If you like that traditional smoky ham flavor in your split pea soup, just stir in 1 teaspoon liquid smoke after the soup comes to a boil. You can find liquid smoke in the spice section of the supermarket."

Hearty Minestrone

Serving Size: 1 cup; Total Servings: 12

3 cans (14 ounces each) reduced-sodium beef broth*

1 can (15-1/2 ounces) red kidney beans, undrained

1 can (15-1/2 ounces) cannellini beans, undrained

1 can (28 ounces) crushed tomatoes

1 package (10 ounces) frozen chopped spinach, thawed

1 package (10 ounces) frozen mixed vegetables, thawed

1 small onion, chopped

1 teaspoon garlic powder*

1/2 teaspoon black pepper

1/2 cup uncooked elbow macaroni*

See photo insert following page 84.

1 In a soup pot, combine all the ingredients except the macaroni. Bring to a boil over medium-high heat then stir in the macaroni.

2 Reduce the heat to low and simmer for 30 minutes, or until the macaroni is tender, stirring occasionally.

*To make this a gluten-free recipe, use gluten-free beef broth; seasoning with no added starch from a gluten-containing source; and quinoa, corn, or brown rice macaroni in place of traditional elbow macaroni.

Exchanges
1 Starch
2 Vegetable

Calories 130
   Calories from Fat 5
Total Fat . . . . 1 g
   Saturated Fat . . . . . . 0.1 g
Cholesterol . . . . 0 mg
Sodium . . . . 602 mg
Total Carbohydrate . . . 24 g
   Dietary Fiber . . . . 6 g
   Sugars . . . . 6 g
Protein . . . . 7 g

Great Go-Along

Using all these convenient ingredients leaves you plenty of time to throw together a fresh Caesar salad and set the table for this simple Italian meal.

Effortless Egg Drop Soup

Serving Size: 1 cup; Total Servings: 7

4 cans (14 ounces each) reduced-sodium chicken broth*

4 tablespoons cornstarch

2 tablespoons light soy sauce*

4 scallions, thinly sliced

2 eggs, lightly beaten

1. In a small bowl, combine 1/2 cup chicken broth and the cornstarch; mix well and set aside.

2. In a soup pot, combine the remaining chicken broth, the soy sauce, and scallions; bring to a boil over high heat.

3. Reduce the heat to low; stir in the cornstarch mixture until the soup is thickened.

4. Slowly stir in the beaten eggs to form egg strands. Ladle into soup bowls and serve.

*To make this a gluten-free recipe, use gluten-free chicken broth and gluten-free soy sauce or pure tamari.

Exchanges
1/2 Carbohydrate

Calories 61
  Calories from Fat . . . 13
Total Fat . . . . 1 g
  Saturated Fat . . . . . . 0.4 g
Cholesterol . . . . 60 mg
Sodium . . . . 736 mg
Total Carbohydrate . . . . 6 g
  Dietary Fiber . . . . 0 g
  Sugars . . . . 1 g
Protein . . . . 5 g

"Next time everybody's in the mood for Chinese take-out, surprise 'em with this homemade version instead. You'll easily reduce the amount of sodium with these lighter ingredients, but you won't lose that classic, restaurant-style taste!"

Vegetarian Onion Soup

Serving Size: 1 cup; Total Servings: 6

Nonstick cooking spray*

3 medium onions, thinly sliced

3 cans (14 ounces each) fat-free, reduced-sodium vegetable broth*

1 cup water

1/2 cup dry red wine

1/2 teaspoon black pepper

6 slices (1/2 ounce each) French bread, toasted*

2 tablespoons grated real Parmesan cheese

1 Coat a soup pot with nonstick cooking spray. Add the onions and sauté over medium heat for 10 to 12 minutes, or until browned.

2 Add the vegetable broth, water, red wine, and pepper; mix well. Reduce the heat to low and simmer for 10 minutes.

3 Ladle soup into bowls and top each with a slice of French bread and a sprinkle of Parmesan cheese. Serve immediately.

*To make this a gluten-free recipe, use nonstick cooking spray with no flour added, gluten-free vegetable broth, and a gluten-free substitute for the French bread.

Exchanges
1/2 Starch
2 Vegetable

Calories	98
Calories from Fat . . .	10
Total Fat	1 g
Saturated Fat	0.4 g
Cholesterol	2 mg
Sodium	414 mg
Total Carbohydrate . . .	18 g
Dietary Fiber	2 g
Sugars	3 g
Protein	3 g

Options

Depending on your meal plan, you can substitute the red wine with cooking sherry or leave it out altogether. Either way, this restaurant favorite will have you crying for joy over the taste . . . not the onions!

Cucumber Gazpacho

Serving Size: 3/4 cup; Total Servings: 4

2 cucumbers, peeled, seeded, and cut into chunks

1/2 cup reduced-sodium chicken broth

1 cup (8 ounces) low-fat plain yogurt

1/8 teaspoon salt

1/8 teaspoon black pepper

1 scallion, thinly sliced

1 In a food processor or blender, combine all the ingredients except the scallion; process until smooth. Cover and chill for at least 2 hours before serving.

2 When ready to serve, ladle soup into bowls and garnish with sliced scallions.

Exchanges
1/2 Carbohydrate

Calories 54
Calories from Fat . . . 10
Total Fat . . . . 1 g
Saturated Fat . . . . . . 0.6 g
Cholesterol . . . . 4 mg
Sodium . . . . 191 mg
Total Carbohydrate . . . . 7 g
Dietary Fiber . . . . 1 g
Sugars . . . . 5 g
Protein . . . . 4 g

Finishing Touch

For a real "ta-da!" factor, add a few very thin slices of cucumber and some diced tomato to each bowl as an additional garnish right before serving.

Rustic White Bean Soup

Serving Size: 1 cup; Total Servings: 8

Nonstick cooking spray*

1/2 pound hot Italian-style turkey sausage, casing removed*

2 medium onions, chopped

2 garlic cloves, minced

2 cans (15-1/2 ounces each) white navy beans, undrained, divided

2 cans (14 ounces each) reduced-sodium chicken broth*

1 package (10 ounces) fresh spinach

1/4 teaspoon black pepper

1 Coat a soup pot with nonstick cooking spray; heat over medium heat.

2 Add the sausage, onions, and garlic and sauté for 8 to 10 minutes, or until the onions are tender and the sausage is no longer pink, stirring to break up the sausage.

3 Mash 1 can of navy beans until smooth. Add to the soup pot along with the chicken broth and the remaining can of whole beans; bring to a boil.

4 Add the spinach and pepper, cover, reduce the heat to low, and simmer for 5 minutes, or until the spinach is wilted. Ladle soup into bowls and serve.

*To make this a gluten-free recipe, use nonstick cooking spray with no flour added, and gluten-free sausage and chicken broth.

Exchanges
1-1/2 Starch
1 Vegetable
1 Lean Meat

Calories 191
  Calories from Fat . . . 24
Total Fat . . . . 3 g
  Saturated Fat . . . . . . 0.7 g
Cholesterol . . . . 14 mg
Sodium . . . . 876 mg
Total Carbohydrate . . . 29 g
  Dietary Fiber . . . . 7 g
  Sugars . . . . 3 g
Protein . . . . 14 g

"Served alongside a crisp salad, this cozy and comforting soup makes a perfect weeknight meal that's sure to draw the family around the dinner table in a flash! Best of all, leftovers are a great next-day lunch."

Turkey Kielbasa Soup

Serving Size: 1 cup; Total Servings: 12

6 medium carrots, peeled and chopped

2 medium onions, chopped

3 cans (14 ounces each) reduced-sodium chicken broth*

2 teaspoons chili powder*

2 teaspoons garlic powder*

1 teaspoon ground thyme*

1/2 teaspoon black pepper

1 package (14 ounces) cooked turkey kielbasa, thinly sliced on the diagonal

2 large tomatoes, coarsely chopped

1 can (15-1/2 ounces) red kidney beans, rinsed and drained

2 cans (16 ounces each) pinto beans, rinsed and drained

1 In a soup pot, combine the carrots, onions, chicken broth, chili powder, garlic powder, thyme, and pepper over medium heat. Cook for 12 to 15 minutes, or until the onions are tender.

2 Add the kielbasa and tomatoes. Reduce the heat to low and simmer for 35 minutes, allowing the flavors to "marry."

3 Add the kidney and pinto beans and cook for 10 minutes. Ladle soup into bowls and serve.

*To make this a gluten-free recipe, use gluten-free chicken broth and seasonings with no added starch from a gluten-containing source.

Exchanges
1-1/2 Starch
1 Vegetable
1 Lean Meat

Calories 197	
Calories from Fat . . . 32	
Total Fat . . . . 4 g	
Saturated Fat . . . . . . 1.2 g	
Cholesterol . . . . 19 mg	
Sodium . . . . 738 mg	
Total Carbohydrate . . . 29 g	
Dietary Fiber . . . . 8 g	
Sugars . . . . 7 g	
Protein . . . . 13 g	

Preparation Tip

To save time during the busy week, make this hearty soup a day in advance and simply reheat it on the stovetop just before serving. Besides saving time, it'll allow all the flavors to mingle overnight so that the soup will taste even better the next day!

Caribbean Fish Chowder

Serving Size: 1 cup; Total Servings: 8

1 teaspoon canola oil

2 ribs celery, chopped

2 medium carrots, chopped

1 large onion, chopped

2 cans (14-1/2 ounces each) diced tomatoes, undrained

2 cans (14 ounces each) reduced-sodium chicken broth*

1 teaspoon dried thyme*

1/4 teaspoon black pepper

1 pound white-fleshed fish, fresh or frozen, cut into 1-inch chunks

1 In a soup pot, heat the oil over medium heat. Add the celery, carrots, and onion and sauté for 10 to 12 minutes, or until the vegetables are tender, stirring frequently.

2 Add the tomatoes, chicken broth, thyme, and pepper and bring to a boil.

3 Add the fish, reduce the heat to low, cover, and simmer for 8 to 10 minutes, or until the fish flakes easily with a fork. Ladle soup into bowls and serve.

*To make this a gluten-free recipe, use gluten-free chicken broth and seasoning with no added starch from a gluten-containing source.

Exchanges
2 Vegetable
1 Lean Meat

Calories 122
   Calories from Fat . . . 27
Total Fat . . . . 3 g
   Saturated Fat . . . . . . 0.1 g
Cholesterol . . . . 22 mg
Sodium . . . . 517 mg
Total Carbohydrate . . . 10 g
   Dietary Fiber . . . . 2 g
   Sugars . . . . 6 g
Protein . . . . 14 g

"Did you know that the ADA recommends that you have two to three servings of fish per week to obtain enough omega-3 fatty acids? In fact, many studies show that foods high in omega-3 fatty acids reduce the risk of heart disease. You can find omega-3 fatty acids in albacore tuna, herring, mackerel, rainbow trout, sardines, salmon, and more, so get creative and make fish in different ways, starting with this yummy chowder!"

Creamy Fish & Veggie Soup

Serving Size: 1 cup; Total Servings: 11

2 cups water, divided

1 can (14 ounces) reduced-sodium chicken broth*

2 pounds white potatoes, peeled and cut into 1/2-inch chunks

1 large onion, chopped

2 ribs celery, chopped

1 carrot, chopped

1 bay leaf

2 cans (12 ounces each) fat-free evaporated milk

4 tablespoons (1/2 stick) light butter

1 pound white-fleshed fish fillets, cut into 1/2-inch chunks

1/2 teaspoon dried thyme*

1/4 teaspoon salt

1/2 teaspoon black pepper

2 tablespoons cornstarch

1 In a soup pot, bring 1-1/2 cups water, the chicken broth, potatoes, onion, celery, carrot, and bay leaf to a boil over high heat.

2 Reduce the heat to medium-low, cover, and simmer for 8 to 10 minutes, or until the vegetables are tender. Add the evaporated milk, butter, fish, thyme, salt, and pepper, and bring to a boil.

3 In a small bowl, whisk the cornstarch and the remaining 1/2 cup water until blended. Add to the soup mixture, stirring until thickened. Remove the bay leaf, ladle soup into bowls, and serve.

*To make this a gluten-free recipe, use gluten-free chicken broth and seasoning with no added starch from a gluten-containing source.

Exchanges

1 Starch
1/2 Fat-Free Milk
1 Vegetable
1 Lean Meat

Calories 197
  Calories from Fat . . . 37
Total Fat . . . . 4 g
  Saturated Fat . . . . . . 1.3 g
Cholesterol . . . . 21 mg
Sodium . . . . 313 mg
Total Carbohydrate . . . 25 g
  Dietary Fiber . . . . 2 g
  Sugars . . . . 9 g
Protein . . . . 15 g

"This rich and hearty cream soup fits right into most any diabetes meal plan because it's a lighter version of the traditional recipe. It brings me back to those cold nights in the Northeast where nothing beats the mid-winter blues better than a warm mug of fill-you-up soup!"

Poultry

Greek Chicken

Serving Size: 1 chicken breast; Total Servings: 6

1 tablespoon vegetable oil

6 boneless, skinless chicken breast cutlets (4 ounces each)

1/2 teaspoon salt

1/4 teaspoon black pepper

1 jar (12 ounces) chicken gravy*

1/4 cup dry white wine

1-1/2 teaspoons fresh lemon juice

1-1/2 teaspoons dried oregano*

2 tablespoons sliced black olives (optional)

1/4 cup crumbled real feta cheese (optional)

See photo insert following page 36.

1 In a large skillet, heat the oil over medium-high heat. Season the chicken with the salt and pepper then brown for 3 to 4 minutes per side.

2 In a small bowl, combine the gravy, wine, lemon juice, and oregano; mix well. Pour over the chicken and simmer for 4 to 5 minutes, or until no pink remains in the chicken. Top with olives and feta cheese, if desired, and serve.

*To make this a gluten-free recipe, use gluten-free gravy and seasoning with no added starch from a gluten-containing source.

Exchanges
4 Very Lean Meat
1 Fat

Calories 176
   Calories from Fat . . . 50
Total Fat . . . . 6 g
   Saturated Fat . . . . . . 1.1 g
Cholesterol . . . . 67 mg
Sodium . . . . 585 mg
Total Carbohydrate . . . . 3 g
   Dietary Fiber . . . . 0 g
   Sugars . . . . 0 g
Protein . . . . 25 g

"This chicken cooks up almost as fast as it gets gobbled up at the dinner table! I like to pair it with steamed broccoli and brown rice for a well-rounded family meal that everybody loves."

Basil- and Cheese-Stuffed Chicken

Serving Size: 1 roll; Total Servings: 4

Nonstick cooking spray*

2 slices (1-1/2 ounces total) fat-free real Swiss cheese, cut in half

4 boneless, skinless chicken breast cutlets (4 ounces each)

8 basil leaves

1 tablespoon olive oil

1 large onion, finely chopped

2 tablespoons white wine

1 Preheat the oven to 350°F. Coat an 8-inch square baking dish with nonstick cooking spray.

2 Place a half-slice of Swiss cheese over each of the chicken breasts. Place 2 basil leaves over each and roll up jelly roll-style; secure each with 2 wooden toothpicks. Place the rolls in the baking dish.

3 In a large skillet, heat the olive oil over medium-high heat. Add the onion and sauté until tender. Add the wine and cook for 2 minutes. Pour over the chicken.

4 Bake for 20 to 25 minutes, or until no pink remains in the chicken.

*To make this a gluten-free recipe, use nonstick cooking spray with no flour added.

Exchanges
1 Vegetable
3 Very Lean Meat
1 Fat

Calories 191
   Calories from Fat . . . 56
Total Fat . . . . 6 g
   Saturated Fat . . . . . . 1.3 g
Cholesterol . . . . 67 mg
Sodium . . . . 124 mg
Total Carbohydrate . . . . 6 g
   Dietary Fiber . . . . 1 g
   Sugars . . . . 3 g
Protein . . . . 26 g

Key West Chicken

Serving Size: 1/4 recipe; Total Servings: 4

2 tablespoons canola oil

1 pound boneless, skinless chicken breast, cut into 1/2-inch strips

1 large red onion, halved and cut into 1/4-inch strips

1 large yellow bell pepper, cut into 1/4-inch strips

1/2 pound asparagus, cut into 2-inch pieces

Juice of 1 orange (about 1/3 cup)

1 tablespoon honey

1 teaspoon garlic powder*

1 teaspoon grated orange peel

1/2 teaspoon salt

1/2 teaspoon black pepper

1 In a large skillet, heat the oil over medium heat. Add the chicken and onion and sauté for 3 to 4 minutes, or until no pink remains in the chicken, stirring occasionally.

2 Add the bell pepper; cover and cook for 3 to 4 minutes.

3 Add the remaining ingredients, cover, and simmer over low heat for 2 to 3 minutes, or until the asparagus is crisp-tender, stirring occasionally. Serve immediately.

*To make this a gluten-free recipe, use seasoning with no added starch from a gluten-containing source.

Exchanges
1/2 Fruit
2 Vegetable
3 Very Lean Meat
1-1/2 Fat

Calories 259
Calories from Fat . . . 88
Total Fat . . . . 10 g
Saturated Fat . . . . . . 1.3 g
Cholesterol . . . . 66 mg
Sodium . . . . 354 mg
Total Carbohydrate . . . 17 g
Dietary Fiber . . . . 2 g
Sugars . . . . 11 g
Protein . . . . 26 g

Finishing Touch

Garnish this tropical chicken with a few slices of lime, just like they do in the free and easy Florida Keys. Then, the next time you're in the mood for a taste of the tropics, try this dish with the catch of the day instead of chicken breast for a fresh change of pace.

All-American Diner Chicken

Serving Size: 1 chicken breast; Total Servings: 6

1/4 cup all-purpose flour*

6 boneless, skinless chicken breast cutlets (4 ounces each)

2 tablespoons olive oil

3 garlic cloves, crushed

2 medium onions, cut in half and sliced

2 medium red bell peppers, cut into 1/2-inch strips

1/2 cup dry white wine

1 chicken bouillon cube*

1 teaspoon dried tarragon*

1/2 teaspoon salt

1/2 teaspoon black pepper

1 Place the flour in a shallow dish. Coat the chicken with flour.

2 In a large nonstick skillet, heat the olive oil over medium-high heat. Add the chicken and cook for 3 to 4 minutes per side, or until golden. Remove the chicken to a platter; set aside.

3 Add the garlic, onions, and bell peppers to the skillet and sauté for 5 to 8 minutes, until the peppers are crisp-tender.

4 Return the chicken to the skillet, and spoon the vegetables over it. Add the wine, bouillon, tarragon, salt, and black pepper; stir until the bouillon is dissolved.

5 Cover and cook over low heat for 18 to 20 minutes, or until no pink remains in the chicken. Serve topped with the vegetables and sauce.

*To make this a gluten-free recipe, use tapioca flour instead of all-purpose flour, gluten-free bouillon, and seasoning with no added starch from a gluten-containing source.

Exchanges
2 Vegetable
3 Very Lean Meat
1-1/2 Fat

Calories 230
  Calories from Fat . . . 68
Total Fat . . . . 8 g
  Saturated Fat . . . . . . 1.4 g
Cholesterol . . . . 66 mg
Sodium . . . . 410 mg
Total Carbohydrate . . . 13 g
  Dietary Fiber . . . . 2 g
  Sugars . . . . 5 g
Protein . . . . 26 g

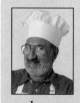

"Bet you never thought you could enjoy this long-cooked taste in a dish you made at home! You can, and in much less time than you thought it would take!"

Asian Chicken Wraps

Serving Size: 1 wrap; Total Servings: 4

2 cups cooked and chunked boneless, skinless chicken breast (see Tips, page 40)

1/2 of a 16-ounce package coleslaw mix (4 cups)

1/2 cup fat-free sesame dressing

1 teaspoon ground ginger

4 eight-inch flour tortillas (see Note)

1 In a large bowl, combine the chicken, coleslaw mix, dressing, and ginger; mix well.

2 Place equal amounts of the chicken mixture onto the center of each tortilla. Wrap each tortilla by folding the bottom over the filling then folding in the right and left sides of the tortilla, forming an envelope. Roll up and place seam-side down on a serving platter. Serve immediately.

Exchanges

1-1/2 Starch
1 Vegetable
3 Very Lean Meat
1 Fat

Calories 317
  Calories from Fat ... 61
Total Fat .... 7 g
  Saturated Fat ...... 1.7 g
Cholesterol .... 72 mg
Sodium .... 576 mg
Total Carbohydrate ... 30 g
  Dietary Fiber .... 3 g
  Sugars .... 5 g
Protein .... 32 g

"I'm a huge fan of Asian cuisine, but when you're watching what you eat, it's sometimes hard to figure out what's actually in your meal—unless you've made it yourself. That's why I love these adorable wraps! Bundle the mixture inside the tortillas or, for a change of pace and fewer carbs, stuff it inside large, crisp Boston lettuce leaves. Talk about refreshing!"

Chicken Rice Skillet

Serving Size: 1-1/4 cups; Total Servings: 5

1 tablespoon olive oil

2 ribs celery, chopped

1 onion, chopped

2 garlic cloves, chopped

1-1/4 pounds boneless skinless chicken breast, cut into 1/2-inch chunks

1/4 pound fresh mushrooms, sliced

2 tablespoons all-purpose flour*

1 cup reduced-sodium chicken broth*

1-1/2 cups low-fat milk

2 cups cooked natural brown rice

1 cup frozen peas, thawed

1 can (8 ounces) water chestnuts, drained

1/2 teaspoon dried tarragon*

1/4 teaspoon salt

1/2 teaspoon black pepper

1 In a large skillet, heat the oil over medium heat. Add the celery, onion, and garlic and sauté for 3 to 5 minutes or until tender.

2 Add the chicken and mushrooms and sauté for 5 minutes, or until the chicken is browned. Sprinkle with flour and stir for 1 minute or until absorbed.

3 Add the chicken broth and milk and cook over medium heat for 5 to 6 minutes, or until the chicken is tender and the sauce is thickened, stirring occasionally.

4 Add the rice, peas, water chestnuts, tarragon, salt, and pepper and cook for 3 to 4 minutes, or until heated through. Serve.

*To make this a gluten-free recipe, use tapioca flour instead of all-purpose flour, gluten-free chicken broth, and seasoning with no added starch from a gluten-containing source.

Exchanges
2 Starch
2 Vegetable
3 Very Lean Meat
1 Fat

Calories 349
   Calories from Fat . . . 65
Total Fat . . . . 7 g
   Saturated Fat . . . . . . 1.8 g
Cholesterol . . . . 70 mg
Sodium . . . . 365 mg
Total Carbohydrate . . . 38 g
   Dietary Fiber . . . . 5 g
   Sugars . . . . 9 g
Protein . . . . 32 g

"There's no need to avoid rice in a diabetes meal plan, especially brown rice. It's quite nutritious, since it's the whole grain of rice, with the germ and outer layers (containing the bran) still intact."

Lemon-Dill Chicken

Serving Size: 3 strips; Total Servings: 4

2 tablespoons all-purpose flour*

1/8 teaspoon salt

1/8 teaspoon black pepper

1 pound boneless, skinless chicken breast, cut into 12 strips

1-1/2 tablespoons olive oil

2 garlic cloves, chopped

1/3 cup reduced-sodium chicken broth*

1/3 cup dry white wine

1 tablespoon fresh lemon juice

1 tablespoon small capers

1 tablespoon chopped fresh dill weed

1 In a shallow dish, combine the flour, salt, and pepper; mix well. Dip the chicken in the seasoned flour until lightly coated.

2 In a large skillet, heat the oil over medium heat. Add the chicken and cook for 2 to 3 minutes per side, until browned. Remove the chicken from the skillet; set aside.

3 Add the garlic to the skillet and sauté for 1 to 2 minutes; add the chicken broth, wine, lemon juice, and capers. Bring to a boil and stir until the sauce is thickened.

4 Return the chicken to the skillet, add the dill, and cook until no pink remains in the chicken. Serve immediately.

*To make this a gluten-free recipe, use tapioca flour instead of all-purpose flour, and gluten-free chicken broth.

Exchanges
4 Very Lean Meat
1 Fat

Calories 198
　Calories from Fat . . . 71
Total Fat . . . . 8 g
　Saturated Fat . . . . . . 1.5 g
Cholesterol . . . . 66 mg
Sodium . . . . 240 mg
Total Carbohydrate . . . . 4 g
　Dietary Fiber . . . . 0 g
　Sugars . . . . 1 g
Protein . . . . 25 g

"Protein is an important part of just about any diet, and the ADA recommends that it make up 15 to 20% of our calories. That's no problem when you have dishes as zesty and flavorful as this one! We enjoy it for dinner and use any leftovers to top a garden salad for lunch the next day. You should too!"

American Pie Chicken

Serving Size: 1 chicken breast; Total Servings: 4

Nonstick cooking spray*

4 boneless, skinless chicken breast cutlets (4 ounces each)

1/2 teaspoon salt

1/8 teaspoon black pepper

1/4 cup apple butter (see Tip)

1/4 cup (1 ounce) shredded, reduced-fat real Cheddar cheese

1 Preheat the oven to 350°F. Coat a 7" x 11" baking dish with nonstick cooking spray.

2 Place the chicken in the baking dish; season the chicken with salt and pepper then spread apple butter evenly over it.

3 Cover with aluminum foil and bake for 25 to 30 minutes, or until no pink remains in the chicken.

4 Remove the baking dish from the oven, uncover, and sprinkle the chicken evenly with cheese. Return the chicken to the oven and bake uncovered for 4 to 6 minutes, or until the cheese is melted.

*To make this a gluten-free recipe, use nonstick cooking spray with no flour added.

Exchanges
1/2 Carbohydrate
4 Very Lean Meat

Calories 173
   Calories from Fat . . . 35
Total Fat . . . . 4 g
   Saturated Fat . . . . . . 1.4 g
Cholesterol . . . . 70 mg
Sodium . . . . 395 mg
Total Carbohydrate . . . . 8 g
   Dietary Fiber . . . . 0 g
   Sugars . . . . 6 g
Protein . . . . 25 g

Tip

Apple butter can be found in the jelly and jam section of your supermarket. Contrary to its name, it does not contain butter . . . but it IS spreadable.

Sun-Dried Tomato Chicken

Serving Size: 1 chicken breast; Total Servings: 4

Nonstick cooking spray*

1 package (10 ounces) fresh spinach

4 bone-in chicken breast halves, with skin removed (8 ounces each)

1 ounce sun-dried tomatoes (6 to 8)

1/2 cup fresh basil leaves

1/4 cup shelled walnuts

1-1/3 tablespoons olive oil

2 garlic cloves

1/8 teaspoon salt

1/8 teaspoon black pepper

1 tablespoon grated real Parmesan cheese (optional)

1 Preheat the oven to 350°F. Coat a 9" x 13" baking dish with non-stick cooking spray; distribute the spinach over the bottom of the baking dish and arrange the chicken over the spinach.

2 In a food processor, process the remaining ingredients, except the Parmesan cheese, until smooth. Spread the mixture evenly over the chicken breasts.

3 Cover and bake for 45 to 50 minutes, or until no pink remains in the chicken. Sprinkle with Parmesan cheese, if desired, and serve.

---

*To make this a gluten-free recipe, use nonstick cooking spray with no flour added.

Exchanges
2 Vegetable
5 Lean Meat

Calories 333
   Calories from Fat . . 129
Total Fat . . . . 14 g
   Saturated Fat . . . . . . 2.4 g
Cholesterol . . . . 107 mg
Sodium . . . . 227 mg
Total Carbohydrate . . . . 8 g
   Dietary Fiber . . . . 3 g
   Sugars . . . . 3 g
Protein . . . . 43 g

"Whether you're cooking for four or fourteen, this elegant-yet-easy recipe is perfect for a quick week-night supper or a fancy dinner party. Because the ingredients are things we generally have on hand, we can double or triple the recipe with ease."

In-a-Hurry Curried Chicken

Serving Size: 1 chicken breast; Total Servings: 4

Nonstick cooking spray*

1 teaspoon canola oil

1 tablespoon chopped fresh parsley

1-1/2 teaspoons curry powder*

1 teaspoon onion powder*

1 teaspoon ground cumin*

1/4 teaspoon black pepper

1/2 teaspoon salt

4 bone-in chicken breast halves, skin removed (8 ounces each)

1 Preheat the oven to 350°F. Coat a rimmed baking sheet with nonstick cooking spray.

2 In a small bowl, combine the oil, parsley, curry powder, onion powder, cumin, and pepper; mix well. Rub the chicken pieces with the seasoning mixture then sprinkle with salt and place on the baking sheet.

3 Bake for 20 to 25 minutes, or until no pink remains in the chicken. Serve immediately.

*To make this a gluten-free recipe, use nonstick cooking spray with no flour added, and seasonings with no added starch from a gluten-containing source.

Exchanges
5 Very Lean Meat
1 Fat

Calories 222
   Calories from Fat . . . 52
Total Fat . . . . 6 g
   Saturated Fat . . . . . . 1.4 g
Cholesterol . . . . 105 mg
Sodium . . . . 385 mg
Total Carbohydrate . . . . 1 g
   Dietary Fiber . . . . 0 g
   Sugars . . . . 0 g
Protein . . . . 39 g

Did You Know . . .

that curry powder, which has been long associated with Indian cooking, is actually made up of around twenty different herbs, spices, and seeds? That makes it a pretty complicated flavoring, one that works just perfectly in here.

Herb-Crusted Chicken

Serving Size: 2 pieces; Total Servings: 5

Nonstick cooking spray*

1/2 cup Panko (Japanese) bread crumbs*

2 tablespoons dried basil*

2 tablespoons dried oregano*

1 teaspoon ground thyme*

1 teaspoon ground rosemary*

1 teaspoon salt

2 egg whites, slightly beaten

1 chicken (3 pounds), cut into 10 pieces, skin removed**

1 Preheat the oven to 425°F. Coat a rimmed baking sheet with nonstick cooking spray.

2 In a shallow dish, combine the bread crumbs, basil, oregano, thyme, rosemary, and salt. Place the egg whites in another shallow dish. Dip the chicken in the egg whites then in the bread crumb mixture, coating completely. Place the chicken on the baking sheet and coat lightly with nonstick cooking spray.

3 Bake for 40 to 45 minutes, or until no pink remains in the chicken. Serve immediately.

*To make this a gluten-free recipe, use gluten-free bread crumb product, seasonings with no added starch from a gluten-containing source, and nonstick cooking spray with no flour added.
**To get 10 pieces of chicken, cut each breast in half.

Exchanges
1/2 Starch
3 Lean Meat

Calories 203
Calories from Fat . . . 62
Total Fat . . . . 7 g
Saturated Fat . . . . . . 1.9 g
Cholesterol . . . . 78 mg
Sodium . . . . 580 mg
Total Carbohydrate . . . . 6 g
Dietary Fiber . . . . 1 g
Sugars . . . . 0 g
Protein . . . . 28 g

Finishing Touch

Make this a winning presentation by topping the chicken with a sprig of fresh basil and serving it alongside your choice of grilled veggies and a fresh garden salad.

Lemon Roasted Chicken

Serving Size: 2 pieces; Total Servings: 5

Nonstick cooking spray*

1 chicken (3 pounds), cut into
   10 pieces, skin removed (see
   note on page 81)

2 teaspoons dried oregano*

1/4 teaspoon salt

1/4 teaspoon black pepper

3 lemons, thinly sliced

1 medium onion, thinly sliced

1 Preheat the oven to 400°F. Coat a 9" x 13" baking dish with nonstick cooking spray.

2 Place the chicken in the baking dish and sprinkle with oregano, salt, and pepper. Place the lemon slices then the onion slices evenly over the chicken. Tightly cover the baking dish with aluminum foil.

3 Bake for 45 minutes. Uncover and bake for 10 to 15 more minutes, or until no pink remains in the chicken.

*To make this a gluten-free recipe, use nonstick cooking spray with no flour added, and seasoning with no added starch from a gluten-containing source.

Exchanges
1 Vegetable
3 Lean Meat

Calories 186
   Calories from Fat . . . 60
Total Fat . . . . 7 g
   Saturated Fat . . . . . . 1.8 g
Cholesterol . . . . 78 mg
Sodium . . . . 193 mg
Total Carbohydrate . . . . 6 g
   Dietary Fiber . . . . 2 g
   Sugars . . . . 2 g
Protein . . . . 26 g

Finishing Touch

How about garnishing each serving with a sprinkle of fresh chopped parsley and a slice of fresh lemon? It'll make this tasty bird look so sensational, it's sure to go flying off your family's dinner plates!

Classic Chicken in a Pot

Serving Size: 2 pieces chicken, 1 cup soup; Total Servings: 5

1 chicken (3 pounds), cut into 10 pieces, skin removed (see note on page 81)

6 medium carrots, peeled and cut into 1-inch pieces

4 ribs celery, cut into 1-inch pieces

2 medium onions, cut into 8 wedges each

5 cups water

1 chicken bouillon cube*

1/2 teaspoon salt

1/2 teaspoon black pepper

1 In a soup pot, combine all the ingredients and bring to a boil over high heat.

2 Reduce the heat to medium-low, cover, and cook for 1 hour, or until the chicken is fall-apart tender. Ladle into bowls and serve.

*To make this a gluten-free recipe, use gluten-free bouillon.

Exchanges
3 Vegetable
3 Lean Meat

Calories 228
Calories from Fat . . . 61
Total Fat . . . . 7 g
Saturated Fat . . . . . . 1.8 g
Cholesterol . . . . 78 mg
Sodium . . . . 571 mg
Total Carbohydrate . . . 14 g
Dietary Fiber . . . . 4 g
Sugars . . . . 7 g
Protein . . . . 27 g

Preparation Tip

You can add other vegetables like potatoes, zucchini, or even garbanzo beans (chickpeas) to give this recipe an exciting fresh flavor every time you make it! Just check out what's in your veggie bin and go for the gusto!

Quick-as-a-Wink Pesto Chicken

Serving Size: 1 chicken breast; Total Servings: 4

Nonstick cooking spray*

4 boneless, skinless chicken breast cutlets (4 ounces each)

4 tablespoons prepared pesto sauce

4 slices (3 ounces total) fat-free real mozzarella cheese

See photo, opposite.

1 Coat a large skillet with nonstick cooking spray and heat over medium-high heat.

2 Cook the chicken for 3 to 4 minutes per side, or until browned.

3 Top each chicken breast with 1 tablespoon pesto sauce and 1 slice of mozzarella cheese. Cover and cook for 2 to 3 minutes, or until no pink remains in the chicken. Serve immediately.

*To make this a gluten-free recipe, use nonstick cooking spray with no flour added.

Exchanges
4 Very Lean Meat
1 Fat

Calories 204
  Calories from Fat . . . 63
Total Fat . . . . 7 g
  Saturated Fat . . . . . . 1.5 g
Cholesterol . . . . 70 mg
Sodium . . . . 382 mg
Total Carbohydrate . . . . 1 g
  Dietary Fiber . . . . 0 g
  Sugars . . . . 1 g
Protein . . . . 32 g

Finishing Touch

To really fancy this up, top each serving with thin slices of plum tomato and a sprig of fresh basil.

Quick-as-a-Wink
Pesto Chicken

Grilled Pita Pizzas

Hearty Minestrone

Peach Melba Parfaits

Stuffed Turkey Breast Dinner

Stuffed Turkey Breast Dinner

Serving Size: 1 roll-up; Total Servings: 8

Nonstick cooking spray*

1/2 of an 8-ounce package of herb stuffing cubes*

1/4 cup dried cranberries

1 cup reduced-sodium ready-to-use chicken broth*

8 boneless, skinless turkey breast cutlets (4 ounces each)

1 jar (12 ounces) turkey gravy*

See photo, opposite.

1 Preheat the oven to 350°F. Coat a 9" x 13" baking dish with nonstick cooking spray.

2 In a large bowl, combine the stuffing cubes, dried cranberries, and broth; mix well.

3 Place the turkey cutlets on a work surface and place an equal amount of the stuffing mixture in the center of each. Roll up each cutlet and place seam-side down in the baking dish. Pour gravy over the roll-ups.

4 Cover and bake for 35 to 40 minutes, or until cooked through and no pink remains in the turkey.

*To make this a gluten-free recipe, use nonstick cooking spray with no flour added, gluten-free stuffing cube substitute, and gluten-free chicken broth and gravy.

Exchanges
1 Starch
3 Very Lean Meat

Calories 189
Calories from Fat . . . 19
Total Fat . . . . 2 g
Saturated Fat . . . . . . 0.4 g
Cholesterol . . . . 62 mg
Sodium . . . . 552 mg
Total Carbohydrate . . . 16 g
Dietary Fiber . . . . 1 g
Sugars . . . . 4 g
Protein . . . . 25 g

"This is my favorite way to enjoy the homestyle flavors of Thanksgiving any time of the year . . . without all the traditional fuss! Since these are practically a complete meal by themselves, all you have to add is your favorite veggie and a big appetite!"

Turkey Taco Pie

Serving Size: 1/8 recipe; Total Servings: 8

Nonstick cooking spray*

1 pound ground turkey breast

1 teaspoon ground cumin*

1 can (16 ounces) vegetarian refried beans*

1 cup salsa

2 cups shredded romaine lettuce

1 large tomato, chopped

1/2 cup (2 ounces) shredded real Cheddar cheese

---

*To make this a gluten-free recipe, use nonstick cooking spray with no flour added, seasoning with no added starch from a gluten-containing source, and gluten-free refried beans.

1 Coat a large nonstick skillet with nonstick cooking spray; heat over medium-high heat.

2 Add the turkey breast and ground cumin and cook for 5 to 6 minutes, or until the turkey is no longer pink, stirring to break up the turkey.

3 Stir in the refried beans and salsa; bring to a boil.

4 Reduce the heat to low; simmer for 5 minutes, or until well combined and heated through, stirring frequently.

5 Remove the skillet from the heat, scrape down the sides with a spatula, and spread the mixture evenly in the skillet.

6 Arrange the lettuce, tomato, and Cheddar cheese in concentric circles on top of the turkey mixture; serve immediately.

Exchanges

1/2 Starch
1 Vegetable
2 Very Lean Meat
1/2 Fat

Calories 153
   Calories from Fat . . . 26
Total Fat . . . . 3 g
   Saturated Fat . . . . . . 1.6 g
Cholesterol . . . . 43 mg
Sodium . . . . 487 mg
Total Carbohydrate . . . 12 g
   Dietary Fiber . . . . 4 g
   Sugars . . . . 2 g
Protein . . . . 19 g

"My grandkids love helping me make this quick-and-easy Mexican favorite, because they can get in on the action too. Cooking with kids is a great way to enjoy quality family time—and that's half the reward of preparing healthy meals."

Sicilian Turkey Meatballs

Serving Size: 5 meatballs; Total Servings: 6

1 pound ground turkey breast

1 pound hot Italian turkey sausage, casing removed*

1-1/2 cups shredded wheat cereal, crushed*

2 egg whites

1 jar (26 ounces) light spaghetti sauce, divided*

1 In a large bowl, combine the turkey, sausage, cereal, egg whites, and 1/2 cup spaghetti sauce; mix well.

2 Form mixture into 1-1/2-inch meatballs; place the meatballs in a soup pot.

3 Add the remaining spaghetti sauce. Cover and cook over medium-low heat for 25 to 30 minutes, or until no pink remains in the meatballs. Serve.

*To make this a gluten-free recipe, use gluten-free sausage, gluten-free cereal substitute, and gluten-free spaghetti sauce.

Exchanges
1-1/2 Carbohydrate
3 Lean Meat

Calories 279
   Calories from Fat . . . 64
Total Fat . . . . 7 g
   Saturated Fat . . . . . . 1.9 g
Cholesterol . . . . 84 mg
Sodium . . . . 943 mg
Total Carbohydrate . . . 23 g
   Dietary Fiber . . . . 4 g
   Sugars . . . . 7 g
Protein . . . . 33 g

"Substituting ground turkey for traditional beef makes these meatballs a healthier choice for eating as is or topping a serving of spaghetti. Believe me, with these, a little goes a long way!"

Barbecued Turkey Loaves

Serving Size: 1 mini meat loaf; Total Servings: 6

Nonstick cooking spray

6 tablespoons barbecue sauce, divided

2 tablespoons water

2/3 cup quick-cooking or old-fashioned rolled oats

2 egg whites, lightly beaten

2 teaspoons chili powder

2 teaspoons Worcestershire sauce

1/2 teaspoon salt

1 pound ground turkey breast

1 small onion, finely chopped

1/2 red or green bell pepper, chopped

1 Preheat the oven to 375°F. Coat a 9" x 13" baking dish with nonstick cooking spray.

2 In a large bowl, combine 3 tablespoons barbecue sauce and the water. Add the oats, egg whites, chili powder, Worcestershire sauce, and salt; mix well. Add the turkey, onion, and bell pepper; mix well.

3 Form the mixture into six oval-shaped meat loaves and place in the baking dish; bake for 30 minutes.

4 Spread the remaining 3 tablespoons barbecue sauce over the tops and bake for 5 more minutes, or until the meat loaves are cooked through and the juices run clear.

Exchanges
1 Carbohydrate
2 Very Lean Meat

Calories 150
   Calories from Fat . . . 14
Total Fat . . . . 2 g
   Saturated Fat . . . . . . 0.3 g
Cholesterol . . . . 47 mg
Sodium . . . . 408 mg
Total Carbohydrate . . . 11 g
   Dietary Fiber . . . . 2 g
   Sugars . . . . 4 g
Protein . . . . 22 g

Options

Switch up the taste each time you make these by using a different brand or flavor of barbecue sauce—smoky one time, zesty the next, and so on!

Snappy Turkey Chili

Serving Size: 1 cup; Total Servings: 8

Nonstick cooking spray*

1 pound ground turkey breast

1 medium onion, chopped

1 medium-sized green bell pepper, chopped

1/2 teaspoon minced garlic

3 cans (16 ounces each) navy beans, rinsed and drained

1 can (28 ounces) whole tomatoes, coarsely chopped

1 cup salsa

2 tablespoons chili powder*

1 teaspoon ground cumin*

1 teaspoon black pepper

1 Coat a soup pot with nonstick cooking spray; heat over medium-high heat. Add the turkey, onion, bell pepper, and garlic. Cook for 5 to 7 minutes, or until the turkey is no longer pink, stirring to break up the turkey.

2 Add the remaining ingredients. Bring to a boil, stirring occasionally.

3 Reduce the heat to low, cover, and simmer for 20 minutes. Ladle into bowls and serve.

---

*To make this a gluten-free recipe, use nonstick cooking spray with no flour added, and seasonings with no added starch from a gluten-containing source.

Exchanges

2 Starch
2 Vegetable
2 Very Lean Meat

Calories 274	
Calories from Fat . . . 15	
Total Fat . . . . 2 g	
Saturated Fat . . . . . . 0.2 g	
Cholesterol . . . . 35 mg	
Sodium . . . . 689 mg	
Total Carbohydrate . . . 41 g	
Dietary Fiber . . . . 10 g	
Sugars . . . . 8 g	
Protein . . . . 26 g	

Finishing Touch

For added flavor and to give this a finished look, sprinkle each serving with additional chopped onion or top each with a dollop of reduced-fat sour cream or your favorite low-fat shredded cheese.

Blackened Turkey Cutlets

Serving Size: 1 turkey cutlet; Total Servings: 4

2 teaspoons paprika*

1 teaspoon crushed dried thyme*

1/2 teaspoon sugar

1/2 teaspoon onion powder*

1/2 teaspoon garlic powder*

1/2 teaspoon salt

1/2 teaspoon black pepper

1/4 teaspoon ground red pepper*

4 boneless, skinless turkey breast cutlets (4 ounces each)

1 In a small bowl, combine all the ingredients except the turkey; mix well. Rub the turkey cutlets well with the seasoning mixture.

2 Heat a large nonstick skillet over high heat.

3 Add the turkey and cook for 2 minutes per side, or until no pink remains. Serve immediately.

*To make this a gluten-free recipe, use seasonings with no added starch from a gluten-containing source.

Exchanges
3 Very Lean Meat

Calories 108
  Calories from Fat 7
Total Fat . . . . .1 g
  Saturated Fat . . . . . . 0.2 g
Cholesterol . . . . 61 mg
Sodium . . . . 330 mg
Total Carbohydrate . . . . 2 g
  Dietary Fiber . . . . 0 g
  Sugars . . . . 1 g
Protein . . . . 22 g

"It doesn't get much easier than this! With just a sprinkling of a few herbs and spices, this turkey goes from ho-hum to WOW in a matter of minutes. Now's that's what I like to call 'fast food!'"

Anytime Turkey Tenders

Serving Size: 1 cup; Total Servings: 5

1 teaspoon canola oil

1 pound boneless, skinless turkey breast, cut into 1" x 2" strips

2 medium onions, thinly sliced

1/2 pound fresh mushrooms, sliced

1 garlic clove, minced

1/2 cup water

1/4 cup dry red wine

2 teaspoons browning and seasoning sauce

1/2 teaspoon salt

1/2 teaspoon black pepper

1 In a large skillet, heat the oil over medium-high heat. Add the turkey and sauté for 4 to 5 minutes, or until lightly browned. Add the onions, mushrooms, and garlic and sauté for 2 to 3 minutes, or until the onions are tender.

2 Reduce the heat to low and add the remaining ingredients. Cook for 2 to 3 minutes, or until heated through, stirring frequently. Serve immediately.

Exchanges
2 Vegetable
2 Very Lean Meat

Calories	135
Calories from Fat	14
Total Fat	2 g
Saturated Fat	0.2 g
Cholesterol	49 mg
Sodium	271 mg
Total Carbohydrate	10 g
Dietary Fiber	1 g
Sugars	4 g
Protein	19 g

Did You Know . . .

that a typical turkey contains about 70% white meat and 30% dark? White meat is a heart-healthy food that contains less fat and fewer calories than dark meat. That doesn't mean we can never have dark meat. Just remember: everything in moderation.

Turkey Cacciatore

Serving Size: 1 cup; Total Servings: 6

1 tablespoon olive oil

2 bell peppers (1 red and 1 green), thinly sliced

1 large onion, halved and cut into 1/4-inch slices

1/4 pound fresh mushrooms, sliced

1-1/2 pounds boneless, skinless turkey breast, cut into 1/2-inch strips

1 jar (26 ounces) light spaghetti sauce*

1/2 cup water

1/4 teaspoon crushed red pepper*

1/4 teaspoon black pepper

1 In a soup pot, heat the oil over medium-high heat. Add the bell peppers, onion, and mushrooms and sauté for 4 to 5 minutes or until tender. Remove from the pot and set aside.

2 Add the turkey to the pot and sauté for 4 to 5 minutes, until browned.

3 Return the vegetables to the pot and add the spaghetti sauce, water, crushed red pepper, and black pepper; mix well. Reduce the heat to medium-low and cook for 10 to 12 minutes, or until the turkey is tender and cooked through, stirring occasionally. Serve immediately.

*To make this a gluten-free recipe, use gluten-free spaghetti sauce, and seasoning with no added starch from a gluten-containing source.

Exchanges
3 Vegetable
3 Very Lean Meat
1/2 Fat

Calories 200
   Calories from Fat . . . 36
Total Fat . . . . 4 g
   Saturated Fat . . . . . . 0.7 g
Cholesterol . . . . 61 mg
Sodium . . . . 627 mg
Total Carbohydrate . . . 17 g
   Dietary Fiber . . . . 4 g
   Sugars . . . . 10 g
Protein . . . . 25 g

"This one-pot wonder is a lifesaver when you need to get a hearty, full-flavored meal on the table in little time. It's jam-packed with tender cuts of turkey and good-for-you veggies that are sure to satisfy everyone's tummy. I like to serve this up with a tossed green salad and sometimes even a thin slice of bread to dip in the mouthwatering sauce."

Bow Ties with Turkey Sausage

Serving Size: 1-1/2 cups; Total Servings: 6

1 package (12 ounces) bow tie pasta (farfalle)*

2 tablespoons olive oil, divided

1 medium onion, diced

1 pound Italian turkey sausage, cut into 1/2-inch slices*

1 can (14-1/2 ounces) diced tomatoes

1 teaspoon dried basil*

1 teaspoon dried thyme*

1 Cook the pasta according to the package directions; drain and set aside.

2 In the same pot, heat 1 tablespoon olive oil over medium heat. Add the onion and sausage and sauté until the onion is tender and the sausage is browned.

3 Add the tomatoes, basil, and thyme and cook for 2 to 3 minutes.

4 Return the pasta to the pot, add the remaining 1 tablespoon olive oil, and stir until the mixture is well combined and heated through. Serve immediately.

*To make this a gluten-free recipe, use a gluten-free pasta (other shapes will work fine), gluten-free sausage, and seasonings with no added starch from a gluten-containing source.

Exchanges

3 Starch
1 Vegetable
1 Lean Meat
1-1/2 Fat

Calories 394
  Calories from Fat . . 123
Total Fat . . . . 14 g
  Saturated Fat . . . . . . 3.3 g
Cholesterol . . . . 48 mg
Sodium . . . . 858 mg
Total Carbohydrate . . . 54 g
  Dietary Fiber . . . . 4 g
  Sugars . . . . 8 g
Protein . . . . 19 g

"It's okay to indulge once in a while, so when I feel like enjoying a serving of pasta, I toss up this easy dish. And just as Mr. Food always suggests, I change up even my favorite dishes now and then, adding different veggies or herbs for a different flavor each time. That's what makes cooking fun and sitting down to dinner so exciting!"

Meats

Sizzlin' Beef Stir-Fry

Serving Size: 1-1/4 cups; Total Servings: 6

1 tablespoon sesame oil

1-1/2 pounds beef flank steak, cut into thin strips

1/2 pound fresh snow peas

1 large red bell pepper, cut into 1/4-inch strips

2 tablespoons minced garlic

1 tablespoon grated fresh ginger

3 tablespoons light soy sauce*

1/2 teaspoon black pepper

2 tablespoons toasted sesame seeds (see Tip)

1 In a large skillet, heat the oil over medium heat. Add the steak strips; sauté for 2 to 3 minutes, or until browned. Remove the steak; set aside.

2 Add the snow peas, bell pepper, garlic, and ginger to the skillet; sauté for 4 to 5 minutes, or until the vegetables are tender.

3 Add the soy sauce, black pepper, and sesame seeds to the skillet; return the steak to the skillet. Simmer for 2 to 3 minutes, stirring until completely mixed and heated through.

*To make this a gluten-free recipe, use gluten-free soy sauce or pure tamari.

Exchanges
1 Vegetable
3 Lean Meat
1/2 Fat

Calories 220
  Calories from Fat . . . 89
Total Fat . . . . 10 g
  Saturated Fat . . . . . . 3.0 g
Cholesterol . . . . 39 mg
Sodium . . . . 336 mg
Total Carbohydrate . . . . 7 g
  Dietary Fiber . . . . 2 g
  Sugars . . . . 4 g
Protein . . . . 25 g

Preparation Tip

Toast the sesame seeds by placing them in a small nonstick skillet over low heat for 3 to 4 minutes, or until golden, turning frequently. Just watch them carefully, and it's as easy as 1-2-3!

Asian Sesame Steak

Serving Size: 3 to 4 slices; Total Servings: 8

3 tablespoons olive oil

2 tablespoons light soy sauce*

1 scallion, thinly sliced

2 garlic cloves, minced

1 tablespoon fresh ginger, minced

1 teaspoon black pepper

1-1/2 pounds beef flank steak, about 1 inch thick

1 tablespoon sesame seeds

---

*To make this a gluten-free recipe, use gluten-free soy sauce or pure tamari.

1 In a large resealable plastic storage bag, combine all the ingredients except the steak and sesame seeds; mix well.

2 Score the steak on both sides by making shallow diagonal cuts 1-1/2 inches apart. Place the steak in the storage bag, seal, and marinate in the refrigerator for at least 4 hours or overnight, turning the bag occasionally.

3 Heat a large grill pan or skillet over high heat until hot. Remove the steak from the marinade and place on the pan, discarding the excess marinade. Cook the steak for 5 to 6 minutes per side for medium-rare, or to desired doneness.

4 Thinly slice the steak across the grain. Sprinkle with sesame seeds and serve.

Exchanges
3 Lean Meat

Calories	151
Calories from Fat	75
Total Fat	8 g
Saturated Fat	2.4 g
Cholesterol	29 mg
Sodium	130 mg
Total Carbohydrate	1 g
Dietary Fiber	0 g
Sugars	0 g
Protein	17 g

"As with many of my other marinated dishes, this one can also be prepared the night before, so it's ready and waiting for you to cook the next day. Besides, the longer you marinate your meats (as long as it's no more than 24 hours), the more flavorful and tender they become. Talk about a real timesaver!"

Kung Pao Beef

Serving Size: 1/8 recipe; Total Servings: 8

1/4 cup light teriyaki sauce*

1 tablespoon cornstarch

1 teaspoon crushed red pepper*

1/2 teaspoon ground ginger*

1-1/2 pounds beef flank steak, thinly sliced

1 tablespoon vegetable oil

1/3 cup dry-roasted, unsalted peanuts

4 scallions, thinly sliced

See photo insert following page 36.

1 In a large bowl, combine the teriyaki sauce, cornstarch, crushed red pepper, and ginger. Add the steak; toss to coat.

2 In a large skillet or wok, heat the oil over high heat.

3 Add the steak mixture; cook for 5 to 7 minutes, or until the steak is cooked through, stirring constantly.

4 Sprinkle with peanuts and scallions and serve.

*To make this a gluten-free recipe, use gluten-free teriyaki sauce and seasonings with no added starch from a gluten-containing source.

Exchanges

3 Lean Meat

Calories 177
  Calories from Fat . . . 83
Total Fat . . . . 9 g
  Saturated Fat . . . . . . 2.4 g
Cholesterol . . . . 29 mg
Sodium . . . . 196 mg
Total Carbohydrate . . . . 4 g
  Dietary Fiber . . . . 1 g
  Sugars . . . . 2 g
Protein . . . . 19 g

"Why call for take-out when you can make your own? And since we can control what goes into our own homemade dish, there's no guesswork involved with this one!"

Sicilian Beef One-Pot

Serving Size: 1 cup; Total Servings: 6

1 tablespoon olive oil

1 pound beef flank steak, trimmed and thinly sliced

2 bell peppers (1 red and 1 green), thinly sliced

1 large onion, cut into wedges

1/2 pound sliced mushrooms

1 jar (26 ounces) light spaghetti sauce*

1/2 cup water

1 In a soup pot, heat the olive oil over medium-high heat. Add the steak; sauté for 6 to 8 minutes, until browned.

2 Add the bell peppers, onion, and mushrooms; sauté for 8 to 10 minutes, or until the vegetables are just tender.

3 Add the spaghetti sauce and water; mix well. Reduce the heat to medium-low, cover, and cook for 45 minutes, or until the steak is tender.

*To make this a gluten-free recipe, use gluten-free spaghetti sauce.

Exchanges
1 Carbohydrate
1 Vegetable
2 Lean Meat

Calories 205
Calories from Fat . . . 67
Total Fat . . . . 7 g
Saturated Fat . . . . . . 2.1 g
Cholesterol . . . . 26 mg
Sodium . . . . 629 mg
Total Carbohydrate . . . 18 g
Dietary Fiber . . . . 4 g
Sugars . . . . 10 g
Protein . . . . 18 g

"Fast, flavorful, and filling, this easy one-pot is a meal in itself! But if you'd like, serve it up with a garden salad or a steamed green veggie and get ready for a true homestyle feast!"

Caramelized Onion Roast

Serving Size: 2 to 3 slices; Total Servings: 8

1 tablespoon canola oil

One 2-1/2-pound beef bottom round roast

1 large red onion, cut into 1/2-inch slices

1 can (14 ounces) reduced-sodium beef broth*

1/4 cup red wine

3 garlic cloves, minced

1/2 teaspoon dried tarragon*

1/2 teaspoon black pepper

1 In a large soup pot, heat the oil over medium heat. Add the roast; cook for 5 to 6 minutes, until brown on all sides. Remove the roast; set aside.

2 Add the onion; cook for 10 to 12 minutes, or until caramelized and brown.

3 Return the roast to the pot. Add the remaining ingredients, cover, and reduce the heat to medium-low. Simmer for 1-1/2 hours, or until the roast is tender. Slice and serve.

*To make this a gluten-free recipe, use gluten-free beef broth and seasoning with no added starch from a gluten-containing source.

Exchanges
4 Lean Meat

Calories 225
Calories from Fat . . . 78
Total Fat . . . . 9 g
Saturated Fat . . . . . . 2.5 g
Cholesterol . . . . 94 mg
Sodium . . . . 132 mg
Total Carbohydrate . . . . 3 g
Dietary Fiber . . . . 0 g
Sugars . . . . 2 g
Protein . . . . 31 g

Did You Know . . .

that bottom round roast is a lean meat that's an excellent source of many vitamins and minerals, including vitamins B6 and B12, iron, riboflavin, and phosphorus? And since it's available at most supermarkets at reasonable prices, it can easily feed your gang for a small price.

Slow-and-Easy Roast

Serving Size: 2 to 3 slices; Total Servings: 8

1 tablespoon canola oil

One 2-pound beef bottom round roast

2 medium onions, chopped

1 medium carrot, chopped

3 garlic cloves, chopped

1/2 pound mushrooms, sliced

2 cans (14 ounces each) diced tomatoes

1 bay leaf*

1 teaspoon dried oregano*

1/2 teaspoon salt

1/2 teaspoon black pepper

1 In a soup pot, heat the oil over medium-high heat. Add the roast; cook for 5 to 6 minutes, until brown on all sides. Remove the roast; set aside.

2 Add the onions, carrot, and garlic to the pot; sauté for 4 minutes.

3 Add the mushrooms; cook for 2 to 3 more minutes, or until the vegetables are tender.

4 Return the roast to the pot. Add the remaining ingredients, cover, and reduce the heat to low. Cook for 1-1/2 hours, or until the beef is tender, stirring occasionally. **Remove the bay leaf**, slice, and serve the roast topped with sauce and vegetables.

*To make this a gluten-free recipe, use seasonings with no added starch from a gluten-containing source.

Exchanges
2 Vegetable
3 Lean Meat

Calories	216
Calories from Fat . . .	68
Total Fat	8 g
Saturated Fat	2.1 g
Cholesterol	75 mg
Sodium	383 mg
Total Carbohydrate . . .	11 g
Dietary Fiber	2 g
Sugars	6 g
Protein	26 g

"Even if you've never made a roast before, don't worry! It doesn't get much easier—or more flavor-packed—than this one-pot dish."

Presto Pesto Roast

Serving Size: 2 to 3 slices; Total Servings: 8

Nonstick cooking spray*

1 cup fresh basil leaves

1/4 cup olive oil

1/2 cup sun-dried tomatoes (about 2 ounces), reconstituted

3 garlic cloves

1/4 teaspoon salt

1/4 teaspoon black pepper

One 2-1/2-pound beef eye of round roast

1 Preheat the oven to 350°F. Coat a roasting pan with nonstick cooking spray.

2 In a food processor, process the basil, oil, sun-dried tomatoes, garlic, salt, and pepper until smooth.

3 Place the roast in the pan; spread the tomato-pesto mixture over the entire roast.

4 Cook the roast for 50 to 60 minutes, or until it reaches the desired doneness.

5 Remove the roast to a cutting board. Slice evenly then spoon pan juices over each serving.

*To make this a gluten-free recipe, use nonstick cooking spray with no flour added.

Exchanges
4 Lean Meat

Calories 247
  Calories from Fat . . 102
Total Fat . . . . 11 g
  Saturated Fat . . . . . . 2.5 g
Cholesterol . . . . 60 mg
Sodium . . . . 115 mg
Total Carbohydrate . . . . 3 g
  Dietary Fiber . . . . 1 g
  Sugars . . . . 1 g
Protein . . . . 32 g

Option

Why not try slicing the meat and serving it as an open-faced sandwich? Pair it with some fresh green beans or grilled mixed veggies and "Presto!"—you'll be in and out of the kitchen in a flash!

Classic Beef Stew

Serving Size: 1 cup; Total Servings: 6

3 tablespoons all-purpose flour

1 pound beef stew meat, cut into 1-inch chunks

1 tablespoon olive oil

1 can (8 ounces) tomato sauce

1-1/2 cups water

1 teaspoon dried rosemary

1 teaspoon salt

1/2 teaspoon black pepper

3 medium zucchini, cut into 1/2-inch chunks

6 medium carrots, cut into 1/2-inch chunks

3 medium onions, quartered

1 teaspoon browning and seasoning sauce

1 Place the flour in a shallow dish; add the beef chunks and toss to coat completely.

2 In a soup pot, heat the oil over medium-high heat. Add the beef; sauté for 8 to 10 minutes, until browned on all sides.

3 Add the tomato sauce, water, rosemary, salt, and pepper; mix well and bring to a boil. Reduce the heat to low, cover, and simmer for 1 hour.

4 Add the remaining ingredients, increase the heat to high, and return to a boil. Reduce the heat to low; simmer for 50 to 60 minutes, or until the beef and vegetables are tender, stirring occasionally.

Exchanges
4 Vegetable
2 Lean Meat

Calories	197
Calories from Fat	50
Total Fat	6 g
Saturated Fat	1.3 g
Cholesterol	38 mg
Sodium	697 mg
Total Carbohydrate	23 g
Dietary Fiber	5 g
Sugars	10 g
Protein	15 g

"If you've been craving a cozy, comforting bowl of stew, you won't be disappointed with this. And it's a great dish to make in advance—even portion it into separate containers, if you need to—so you can serve it up any day, any time, anywhere!"

Dijon & Pepper-Crusted Steak

Serving Size: 1 filet; Total Servings: 4

4 filet mignon steaks (4 ounces each), well trimmed

2 tablespoons Dijon mustard

2 teaspoons crushed peppercorns

1 Preheat the grill to medium heat.

2 Heavily coat the top of the filets with half the Dijon mustard then sprinkle with half the crushed peppercorns.

3 Place filets coated-side down on the grill. Coat the other side with the remaining mustard and sprinkle with the remaining peppercorns.

4 Grill for 5 to 6 minutes per side, or until cooked to desired doneness.

Thumbs-up for gluten-free meal plans!

Exchanges

3 Lean Meat

Calories 149
   Calories from Fat . . . 54
Total Fat . . . . 6 g
   Saturated Fat . . . . . . 2.2 g
Cholesterol . . . . 58 mg
Sodium . . . . 223 mg
Total Carbohydrate . . . . 1 g
   Dietary Fiber . . . . 0 g
   Sugars . . . . 0 g
Protein . . . . 21 g

Preparation Tip

Weather not cooperating or you don't have an outdoor grill? No problem! These tender, juicy steaks can also be grilled indoors on a grill pan or cooked right under your broiler.

Fiesta Meat Loaf

Serving Size: 1 slice; Total Servings 8

Nonstick cooking spray*

2 pounds 95–96% lean ground beef

1 can (14-1/2 ounces) Mexican-style stewed tomatoes

1 cup plain bread crumbs*

1 medium onion, finely chopped

1/2 cup egg substitute*

1-1/2 teaspoons ground cumin*

1 teaspoon chili powder* (see Option)

1 garlic clove, minced

1/2 teaspoon salt

1/2 teaspoon black pepper

1. Preheat the oven to 350°F. Coat a 9" x 5" loaf pan with nonstick cooking spray.

2. In a large bowl, combine all the ingredients; mix well. Place the mixture in the prepared loaf pan.

3. Bake for 70 to 75 minutes, or until the juices run clear.

4. Drain off the excess liquid and allow the meat loaf to sit for 15 minutes. Remove the meat loaf to a cutting board and slice. Serve immediately.

*To make this a gluten-free recipe, use nonstick cooking spray with no flour added, a gluten-free bread crumb product, gluten-free egg substitute, and seasonings with no added starch from a gluten-containing source.

Exchanges
1/2 Starch
1 Vegetable
3 Lean Meat

Calories 234
   Calories from Fat . . . 61
Total Fat . . . . 7 g
   Saturated Fat . . . . . . 2.8 g
Cholesterol . . . . 69 mg
Sodium . . . . 455 mg
Total Carbohydrate . . . 15 g
   Dietary Fiber . . . . 2 g
   Sugars . . . . 4 g
Protein . . . . 27 g

Option

Make this spicy or not-so-spicy—it's up to you. Go ahead and add as much chili powder as you'd like or leave it out altogether.

Two-Step Meat Loaf Muffins

Serving Size: 1 mini meat loaf; Total Servings: 6

Nonstick cooking spray*

1 pound 95–96% lean ground beef

1/2 medium zucchini, shredded

1 egg white

1/2 cup plain bread crumbs*

1/2 teaspoon dried Italian seasoning*

1/4 teaspoon salt

4 tablespoons barbecue sauce, divided*

1 Preheat the oven to 400°F. Coat a 6-cup muffin pan with non-stick cooking spray.

2 In a large bowl, combine the beef, zucchini, egg white, bread crumbs, Italian seasoning, salt, and 2 tablespoons barbecue sauce; mix lightly but thoroughly. Divide the beef mixture evenly among the 6 muffin cups. Smooth the tops and spread the remaining 2 tablespoons barbecue sauce over the tops.

3 Bake for 25 to 30 minutes, or until no pink remains and the juices run clear.

*To make this a gluten-free recipe, use nonstick cooking spray with no flour added, a gluten-free bread crumb product, gluten-free barbecue sauce, and seasonings with no added starch from a gluten-containing source.

Exchanges
1/2 Starch
2 Lean Meat

Calories 148
Calories from Fat . . . 41
Total Fat . . . . 5 g
Saturated Fat . . . . . . 1.9 g
Cholesterol . . . . 46 mg
Sodium . . . . 301 mg
Total Carbohydrate . . . . 8 g
Dietary Fiber . . . . 1 g
Sugars . . . . 2 g
Protein . . . . 17 g

Preparation Tip

If your family loves meat loaf, why not give this quick 'n' easy recipe a new taste each time you make it? Try it with hickory-smoked, honey-garlic, and other types of barbecue sauces for different twists!

Guilt-Free Picadillo

Serving Size: 1 cup; Total Servings: 4

1 pound 95–96% lean ground beef

1 medium onion, chopped

1 can (14-1/2 ounces) whole tomatoes, undrained, broken up

1/4 cup chopped pimiento-stuffed olives

1/4 cup raisins*

2 teaspoons chili powder*

1 teaspoon garlic powder*

1/2 teaspoon ground cinnamon*

1/4 teaspoon salt

1/4 teaspoon black pepper

1 In a large skillet, cook the ground beef and onion over medium heat, until browned and no pink remains in the meat.

2 Add the remaining ingredients; mix well. Reduce the heat to low and simmer for 5 minutes, until the mixture is heated through. Serve immediately.

*To make this a gluten-free recipe, use raisins that have not been dusted with wheat flour to prevent sticking, and seasonings with no added starch from a gluten-containing source.

Exchanges
1/2 Fruit
2 Vegetable
3 Lean Meat

Calories 233
   Calories from Fat . . . 67
Total Fat . . . . 7 g
   Saturated Fat . . . . . . 2.9 g
Cholesterol . . . . 69 mg
Sodium . . . . 618 mg
Total Carbohydrate . . . 17 g
   Dietary Fiber . . . . 3 g
   Sugars . . . . 12 g
Protein . . . . 24 g

Serving Tip

To keep the carbs low, simply serve this scooped onto a leaf of Bibb or romaine lettuce.

Mouthwatering Pork Marsala

Serving Size: 2 to 3 slices; Total Servings: 6

1/4 cup all-purpose flour*

1/2 teaspoon salt, divided

1 teaspoon black pepper, divided

1-1/2 pounds center-cut pork loin, cut into 1/4-inch slices, well trimmed

2 tablespoons canola oil, divided

1/2 pound mushrooms, sliced

1 medium onion, chopped

2 garlic cloves, minced

1 small tomato, chopped

1/2 cup reduced-sodium chicken broth*

1/4 cup Marsala wine

---

*To make this a gluten-free recipe, use tapioca flour instead of all-purpose flour and gluten-free chicken broth.

Exchanges
2 Vegetable
3 Lean Meat
1/2 Fat

Calories 241
 Calories from Fat . . 107
Total Fat . . . . 12 g
 Saturated Fat . . . . . . 2.8 g
Cholesterol . . . . 59 mg
Sodium . . . . 275 mg
Total Carbohydrate . . . 10 g
 Dietary Fiber . . . . 1 g
 Sugars . . . . 3 g
Protein . . . . 22 g

1 In a shallow dish, combine the flour, 1/4 teaspoon salt, and 1/2 teaspoon pepper; mix well. Coat the pork in the seasoned flour.

2 In a large skillet, heat 1 tablespoon oil over medium heat. Add the pork; sauté in batches for 1 to 2 minutes per side, adding the remaining oil as necessary. Remove the pork from the skillet; set aside.

3 Add the mushrooms, onion, and garlic to the skillet; sauté for 6 to 8 minutes, until the onion is tender, stirring occasionally.

4 Add the tomato, chicken broth, wine, and the remaining 1/4 teaspoon salt and 1/2 teaspoon pepper. Bring to a boil; boil for 3 to 4 minutes.

5 Return the pork to the skillet; cook for 2 minutes, or until heated through. Serve topped with Marsala sauce.

"Wait 'til you get a load of the heavenly aroma that'll fill your kitchen when you cook up this first-class dish. When you get a craving for mushrooms, onions, and tender pork cooked up in a tempting sauce, put together this restaurant-popular main-dish masterpiece right at home!"

Italian Pork Roast

Serving Size: 2 slices; Total Servings: 6

Nonstick cooking spray*

1/2 teaspoon dried oregano*

1/2 teaspoon dried basil*

1/2 teaspoon onion powder*

1/2 teaspoon garlic powder*

1/4 teaspoon salt

1/2 teaspoon black pepper

One 2-pound boneless center-cut pork loin, well trimmed

1 Preheat the oven to 375°F. Coat a roasting pan with nonstick cooking spray.

2 In a small bowl, combine the oregano, basil, onion powder, garlic powder, salt, and pepper. Rub the seasoning mixture into all sides of the pork roast and place in the roasting pan.

3 Bake for 35 to 40 minutes, or until the juices run clear and the roast is cooked to the desired doneness. Slice and serve.

*To make this a gluten-free recipe, use nonstick cooking spray with no flour added, and seasonings with no added starch from a gluten-containing source.

Exchanges
4 Lean Meat

Calories	204
Calories from Fat	86
Total Fat	10 g
Saturated Fat	3.3 g
Cholesterol	78 mg
Sodium	144 mg
Total Carbohydrate	1 g
Dietary Fiber	0 g
Sugars	0 g
Protein	27 g

"Pork loin is perfect for almost any meal plan— including ones low in carbs, like ours. And it's really versatile, because we can serve it up as an easy weeknight supper or an elegant crowd-pleaser!"

Ginger Pork Tenderloin

Serving Size: 4 to 6 slices; Total Servings: 8

2 tablespoons olive oil

2 tablespoons light soy sauce*

1 tablespoon honey

1 tablespoon grated fresh ginger

3 garlic cloves, chopped

2 pork tenderloins (about
    2 pounds total)

1 tablespoon peanut oil

---

*To make this a gluten-free recipe, use gluten-free soy sauce or pure tamari.

1 In a resealable plastic storage bag or shallow dish, combine the olive oil, soy sauce, honey, ginger, and garlic; add the tenderloins. Seal the bag or cover the dish and marinate the tenderloins in the refrigerator for 30 minutes, turning occasionally.

2 In a large skillet, heat the peanut oil over medium heat. Place the tenderloins in the skillet, reserving the marinade. Cook for 12 to 15 minutes, or until medium doneness, turning to brown all sides.

3 Meanwhile, in a small saucepan, bring the reserved marinade to a boil over high heat; let boil for 5 minutes. Slice the tenderloin and serve topped with the sauce.

Exchanges
3 Lean Meat
1/2 Fat

Calories 194
  Calories from Fat . . . 82
Total Fat . . . . 9 g
  Saturated Fat . . . . . . 2.1 g
Cholesterol . . . . 66 mg
Sodium . . . . 190 mg
Total Carbohydrate . . . . 3 g
  Dietary Fiber . . . . 0 g
  Sugars . . . . 3 g
Protein . . . . 24 g

Great Go-Along

Pair this mouth-watering Asian favorite with wasabi mashed potatoes by adding wasabi (Japanese horseradish) to prepared mashed potatoes. Look for wasabi powder or paste in the ethnic foods section of the supermarket. And remember, because it's extremely fiery, a little wasabi goes a long way.

Pronto Polynesian Pork

Serving Size: 1-1/3 cups; Total Servings: 6

1 tablespoon canola oil

1-1/2 pounds pork tenderloin, cut into 3/4-inch chunks

1 can (20 ounces) chunked pineapple in its own juice, drained with liquid reserved

1 can (8 ounces) sliced water chestnuts, drained

1 cup fresh broccoli florets

1 red bell pepper, cut into 3/4-inch chunks

2 tablespoons light soy sauce*

1 tablespoon white vinegar

1 tablespoon ketchup*

2 tablespoons cornstarch

2 tablespoons sugar

1 In a large skillet or wok, heat the oil over high heat. Add the pork and stir-fry for 4 to 5 minutes, or until no pink remains.

2 Add the pineapple, water chestnuts, broccoli, and bell pepper; stir-fry for 6 to 8 minutes, or until the vegetables are crisp-tender.

3 In a small bowl, combine the reserved pineapple juice, soy sauce, vinegar, ketchup, cornstarch, and sugar; mix well. Stir into the pork and vegetable mixture; cook for 4 minutes. Serve immediately.

*To make this a gluten-free recipe, use gluten-free soy sauce or pure tamari and use gluten-free ketchup.

Exchanges
1-1/2 Fruit
1 Vegetable
3 Lean Meat

Calories 270
  Calories from Fat . . . 58
Total Fat . . . . 6 g
  Saturated Fat . . . . . . 1.6 g
Cholesterol . . . . 66 mg
Sodium . . . . 278 mg
Total Carbohydrate . . . 28 g
  Dietary Fiber . . . . 3 g
  Sugars . . . . 20 g
Protein . . . . 25 g

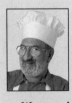

"This flavor paradise is a colorful combination of refreshing fruit, healthy veggies, and tender meat that'll have you feeling like you're sitting down at a luau . . . right at your own table!"

Herb-Crusted Pork Tenderloin

Serving Size: 4 to 6 slices; Total Servings: 6

2 pork tenderloins (about 1-1/4 pounds total)

2 tablespoons water

1 teaspoon browning and seasoning sauce

1 tablespoon chopped fresh parsley

1 teaspoon garlic powder

1/2 teaspoon rubbed sage

1/2 teaspoon salt

1/2 teaspoon black pepper

1 Preheat the oven to 350°F. Place the pork in a 7" x 11" baking dish.

2 In a small bowl, combine the water and browning and seasoning sauce; mix well and then spoon over the pork.

3 In another small bowl, combine the remaining ingredients; mix well then rub evenly over the pork.

4 Bake covered for 25 to 30 minutes, or to desired doneness. Slice and serve with the pan drippings.

Exchanges
2 Lean Meat

Calories	119
Calories from Fat	30
Total Fat	3 g
Saturated Fat	1.2 g
Cholesterol	55 mg
Sodium	235 mg
Total Carbohydrate	1 g
Dietary Fiber	0 g
Sugars	0 g
Protein	20 g

"Nowadays, we can brown our meat in a variety of ways, besides using browning and seasoning sauce. For a tasty change of pace, try light soy or barbecue sauce, low-sugar marmalade, or even brown gravy. Mmm!"

Mojo Pork Grillers

Serving Size: 1 skewer; Total Servings: 6

6 twelve-inch wooden or metal skewers

1/2 cup mojo marinade (see Note)

2 scallions, chopped

2 tablespoons chopped fresh parsley

2 garlic cloves, minced

1 pound boneless pork tenderloin, cut into 12 chunks

1 zucchini, cut into 12 chunks

12 cherry tomatoes

1 If using wooden skewers, soak in water for 15 minutes.

2 In a 9" x 13" baking dish, combine the mojo marinade, scallions, parsley, and garlic; mix well.

3 Alternately skewer 2 chunks of pork, 2 chunks of zucchini, and 2 cherry tomatoes onto each skewer. Place the skewers in the baking dish, turning to coat well. Cover and marinate in the refrigerator for 2 to 3 hours, turning the skewers occasionally.

4 Preheat the grill to medium heat. Grill the skewers for 4 to 5 minutes per side, or until no pink remains in the pork.

Exchanges
1 Vegetable
2 Lean Meat

Calories 116
    Calories from Fat . . . 31
Total Fat . . . . 3 g
    Saturated Fat . . . . . . 1.0 g
Cholesterol . . . . 44 mg
Sodium . . . . 129 mg
Total Carbohydrate . . . . 4 g
    Dietary Fiber . . . . 1 g
    Sugars . . . . 2 g
Protein . . . . 17 g

Did You Know . . .

that mojo (pronounced mo-ho) is a traditional Cuban combination of garlic, citrus juice, and a variety of herbs and spices? Its intense flavor gives just about any type of meat a fun and exciting taste, while remaining low in fat, calories, and carbohydrates!

Honey-Garlic Pork Chops

Serving Size: 1 pork chop; Total Servings: 6

1/4 cup lemon juice

1/4 cup honey

1/4 cup light soy sauce*

1/4 cup dry white wine

2 tablespoons minced garlic

6 boneless pork loin chops, well trimmed (4 ounces each)

1 tablespoon vegetable oil

1 In a 9" x 13" baking dish, combine the lemon juice, honey, soy sauce, wine, and garlic; mix well. Add the pork chops then cover and refrigerate for at least 4 hours or overnight, turning the pork chops occasionally.

2 In a large skillet, heat the oil over medium-high heat.

3 Add the chops; sauté for 2 to 3 minutes per side. Pour the marinade over the chops and bring it to a boil. Reduce the heat to low and simmer for 2 to 3 minutes, or to desired doneness. Serve topped with the sauce.

*To make this a gluten-free recipe, use gluten-free soy sauce or pure tamari.

Exchanges
1 Carbohydrate
3 Lean Meat

Calories 231
  Calories from Fat . . . 85
Total Fat . . . . 9 g
  Saturated Fat . . . . . . 2.7 g
Cholesterol . . . . 59 mg
Sodium . . . . 420 mg
Total Carbohydrate . . . 14 g
  Dietary Fiber . . . . 0 g
  Sugars . . . . 13 g
Protein . . . . 22 g

Finishing Touch

Just before serving, top each chop with a slice of fresh lemon or a sprinkle of chopped scallions.

Rubbed Pork Chops

Serving Size: 1 chop; Total Servings: 4

Nonstick cooking spray*

2 teaspoons ground cumin*

2 teaspoons dried oregano*

2 teaspoons chili powder*

2 teaspoons garlic powder*

4 boneless pork chops
(4 ounces each)

1 Preheat the oven to 375°F. Coat a 9" x 13" baking dish with nonstick cooking spray.

2 In a shallow dish, combine all the ingredients except the pork chops.

3 Rub the seasoning mixture onto both sides of the pork chops and place in the baking dish. Spray the tops of the pork chops with nonstick cooking spray.

4 Bake for 20 to 22 minutes, or until tender and cooked through.

*To make this a gluten-free recipe, use nonstick cooking spray with no flour added, and seasonings with no added starch from a gluten-containing source.

Exchanges
3 Lean Meat

Calories 166
   Calories from Fat . . . 69
Total Fat . . . . 8 g
   Saturated Fat . . . . . . 2.5 g
Cholesterol . . . . 59 mg
Sodium . . . . 51 mg
Total Carbohydrate . . . . 3 g
   Dietary Fiber . . . . 1 g
   Sugars . . . . 1 g
Protein . . . . 21 g

"You know, a spice rub is a really simple way to jazz up meat right before cooking, especially when you don't have time to wait for a marinade to do the job. You can experiment with different herbs and spices to create your own special rubs. Keep your favorite dry blends in spice jars for whenever you need loads of flavor in a hurry!"

Speedy Skillet Veal Française

Serving Size: 1 cutlet; Total Servings: 6

1/2 cup all-purpose flour*

1 tablespoon chopped fresh parsley

1/2 teaspoon salt

3/4 cup egg substitute*

2 tablespoons olive oil

6 boneless veal cutlets (4 ounces each), trimmed of visible fat

1/2 cup dry white wine or vermouth

Juice of 1 lemon

1 In a shallow dish, combine the flour, parsley, and salt; mix well. Place the egg substitute in another shallow dish.

2 In a large skillet, heat the oil over medium heat. Dip the veal in the seasoned flour then in the egg substitute, coating completely.

3 Sauté the veal in batches for 2 to 3 minutes per side, or until golden.

4 Add the wine and lemon juice to the skillet; mix well. Return the veal to the skillet. Cook for 2 to 3 minutes, or until the sauce begins to thicken slightly. Serve veal topped with sauce.

*To make this a gluten-free recipe, use tapioca flour instead of all-purpose flour and gluten-free egg substitute.

Exchanges
1/2 Starch
3 Lean Meat

Calories	236
Calories from Fat . . .	71
Total Fat	8 g
Saturated Fat	1.8 g
Cholesterol	90 mg
Sodium	299 mg
Total Carbohydrate	9 g
Dietary Fiber	0 g
Sugars	1 g
Protein	29 g

Finishing Touch

It's easy to fancy this up! Simply garnish with lemon slices and a sprinkle of fresh chopped parsley and capers just before serving.

Fish & Seafood

Coco-Loco Shrimp

Serving Size: 5 shrimp; Total Servings: 8

Nonstick cooking spray*

1/3 cup cornstarch

1/2 teaspoon ground red pepper*

1/8 teaspoon salt

2 egg whites

1 tablespoon honey

1 tablespoon fresh lime juice

6 tablespoons sweetened flaked coconut, finely chopped

40 large uncooked shrimp (about 1-1/2 pounds), peeled and deveined, tails left on

1 Preheat the oven to 425°F. Coat a baking sheet with nonstick cooking spray.

2 In a small bowl, combine the cornstarch, red pepper, and salt. In another small bowl, whisk together the egg whites, honey, and lime juice. Place the coconut in a shallow dish.

3 Dip the shrimp in the cornstarch mixture then the egg mixture and roll in the coconut, coating completely. Place the shrimp on the baking sheet and lightly spray the tops with nonstick cooking spray.

4 Bake for 10 to 12 minutes, or until the shrimp are pink and the coconut is lightly toasted.

*To make this a gluten-free recipe, use nonstick cooking spray with no flour added, and seasoning with no added starch from a gluten-containing source.

Exchanges
1/2 Carbohydrate
2 Very Lean Meat

Calories 99
 Calories from Fat . . . 15
Total Fat . . . . 2 g
 Saturated Fat . . . . . . 1.1 g
Cholesterol . . . . 98 mg
Sodium . . . . 174 mg
Total Carbohydrate . . . . 9 g
 Dietary Fiber . . . . 0 g
 Sugars . . . . 3 g
Protein . . . . 12 g

"I'm a big fan of 'oven-frying,' and you will be too after you've tried baking these island-style shrimp. No matter how pressed for time you are, it's almost as fast to bake these in the oven as it is to fill your pan with lots of oil and fry them—and it's a lot healthier."

Sweet 'n' Spicy Shrimp

Serving Size: 1 skewer; Total Servings: 4

4 wooden or metal skewers

32 large uncooked shrimp
(about 1 pound), peeled and
deveined, tails left on

1/2 cup sugar-free apricot
preserves

1/4 teaspoon ground red pepper*

1 teaspoon vegetable oil

1/2 teaspoon soy sauce*

See photo insert following page 36.

1 If using wooden skewers, soak them in water for 15 minutes. Preheat the grill to medium-high heat.

2 Thread 8 shrimp on each skewer; set aside.

3 In a small bowl, combine the remaining ingredients. Brush the shrimp skewers with the apricot mixture.

4 Grill the shrimp for 2 to 3 minutes per side, basting with any remaining mixture during grilling. Serve immediately.

*To make this a gluten-free recipe, use seasoning with no added starch from a gluten-containing source and gluten-free soy sauce or pure tamari.

Exchanges
1/2 Carbohydrate
2 Very Lean Meat

Calories 97
  Calories from Fat . . . 17
Total Fat . . . . 2 g
  Saturated Fat . . . . . . 0.3 g
Cholesterol . . . . 131 mg
Sodium . . . . 187 mg
Total Carbohydrate . . . . 5 g
  Dietary Fiber . . . . 0 g
  Sugars . . . . 0 g
Protein . . . . 14 g

Options

*Don't have time to fire
up the grill? No problem!
These shrimp can also be cooked
on an indoor grill, broiled, or
baked just until they
turn pink.*

One-Pot Paella

Serving Size: 1-1/4 cups; Total Servings: 6

Nonstick cooking spray*

1/2 pound turkey sausage, cut into 1/2-inch slices*

1 medium-sized onion, chopped

1 medium-sized red bell pepper, cut into thin strips

3 garlic cloves, minced

1 teaspoon dried thyme*

1-1/2 cups uncooked long-grain rice*

3/4 cup water

1 can (14-1/2 ounces) diced tomatoes, undrained

2 bottles (8 ounces each) clam juice

1/2 teaspoon ground turmeric*

1/2 pound medium shrimp, peeled and deveined

1 Coat a soup pot with nonstick cooking spray. Cook the turkey sausage over medium heat for 4 to 5 minutes, or until browned.

2 Add the onion, bell pepper, garlic, and thyme. Cook for 3 to 5 minutes, or until the vegetables are tender.

3 Add the rice, water, tomatoes and their juice, the clam juice, and turmeric; mix well. Bring to a boil then reduce the heat to low, cover, and simmer for 20 minutes.

4 Stir in the shrimp; cook for 5 minutes, or until the shrimp are pink and cooked through, the rice is tender, and no liquid remains.

*To make this a gluten-free recipe, use nonstick cooking spray with no flour added, gluten-free sausage, seasonings with no added starch from a gluten-containing source, and rice that has not been enriched.

Exchanges
2-1/2 Starch
2 Vegetable
1 Lean Meat

Calories 286
　Calories from Fat . . . 43
Total Fat . . . . 5 g
　Saturated Fat . . . . . . 1.4 g
Cholesterol . . . . 70 mg
Sodium . . . . 716 mg
Total Carbohydrate . . . 48 g
　Dietary Fiber . . . . 3 g
　Sugars . . . . 6 g
Protein . . . . 15 g

"Paella (pronounced pie-ay-yuh) is traditionally made with a variety of meats, shellfish, and veggies, each usually prepared separately before being combined in one pot. My 'light' version is easier, since everything cooks together in one pot."

Snappy Scallop Stir-Fry

Serving Size: 1-1/4 cups; Total Servings: 5

2 tablespoons sesame oil

2 cups broccoli florets

1 medium onion, sliced

1/4 pound fresh snow peas

1/2 large red bell pepper, cut into strips

2 garlic cloves, minced

1 teaspoon fresh grated ginger

1 pound sea scallops

3 cups thinly sliced bok choy

1 cup sliced shiitake mushrooms

1/2 cup low-sodium chicken broth*

1/4 cup rice wine vinegar

3 teaspoons light soy sauce*

2 tablespoons cornstarch

1/4 cup water

1 In a large skillet or wok, heat the sesame oil over medium-high heat. Add the broccoli, onion, snow peas, bell pepper, garlic, and ginger; stir-fry for 3 to 4 minutes.

2 Add the scallops, bok choy, and mushrooms; stir-fry for 3 to 4 minutes.

3 Add the chicken broth, vinegar, and soy sauce. Reduce the heat to medium-low and simmer for 5 minutes, or until the scallops are cooked through and the vegetables are tender.

4 In a small bowl, whisk the cornstarch into the water. Add to the scallop mixture, stirring until the sauce is thickened. Serve immediately.

*To make this a gluten-free recipe, use gluten-free chicken broth and gluten-free soy sauce or pure tamari.

"Stir-frying is an easy way to incorporate a variety of proteins and veggies into your meal plan. I like to experiment with different sauces and spices to give my stir-fry dishes a new flavor each time, but what I really love is that I don't crave the rice most restaurants serve this over. Because it's so hearty and delicious, I don't feel like I'm sacrificing anything!"

Exchanges
3 Vegetable
2 Very Lean Meat
1 Fat

Calories 189
Calories from Fat . . . 62
Total Fat . . . . 7 g
Saturated Fat . . . . . . 0.9 g
Cholesterol . . . . 36 mg
Sodium . . . . 344 mg
Total Carbohydrate . . . 13 g
Dietary Fiber . . . . 3 g
Sugars . . . . 5 g
Protein . . . . 19 g

Lemon Pepper-Crusted Tuna

Serving Size: 1 steak; Total Servings: 4

2 tablespoons lemon juice

1 tablespoon wasabi paste*
(see Note, page 111)

1 teaspoon grated lemon peel

1 teaspoon black peppercorns,
crushed

4 tuna steaks (4 ounces each)

1 In an 8-inch square baking dish, combine the lemon juice, wasabi paste, lemon peel, and crushed peppercorns; add the tuna steaks and marinate for 20 minutes, turning occasionally.

2 Heat a grill pan or skillet over high heat. Place the tuna in the pan and pour the marinade over it.

3 Grill for 2 minutes per side for rare, or to desired doneness. Serve the tuna as is or slice thinly and fan out the slices to give it a fancier presentation.

*To make this a gluten-free recipe, use pure wasabi paste.

Did You Know . . .

that it's easy to tell if tuna is fresh or previously frozen? Fresh tuna steaks are red or pink, without any brown. Cook them for just a few minutes to keep their moist texture and delicate flavor. Sushi grade tuna is the best quality available. When prepared properly, it doesn't taste "fishy," so many people eat it raw or cook it to rare or medium-rare.

Exchanges
3 Lean Meat

Calories 170
   Calories from Fat . . . 52
Total Fat . . . . 6 g
   Saturated Fat . . . . . . 1.5 g
Cholesterol . . . . 42 mg
Sodium . . . . 119 mg
Total Carbohydrate . . . . 3 g
   Dietary Fiber . . . . 0 g
   Sugars . . . . 2 g
Protein . . . . 25 g

Zesty Sesame Tuna Steaks

Serving Size: 1 tuna steak; Total Servings: 2

1/4 cup light soy sauce*

3 teaspoons wasabi paste*
(see Note, page 111)

1/2 teaspoon cracked black pepper

2 Ahi tuna steaks, 3/4 inch thick (4 ounces each)

Nonstick cooking spray*

2 tablespoons sesame seeds

1. In a shallow dish, combine the soy sauce, wasabi paste, and cracked black pepper; mix well. Add the tuna and turn until thoroughly coated on both sides; let sit for 10 minutes.

2. Coat a grill pan with nonstick cooking spray and preheat over high heat.

3. Place the sesame seeds in another shallow dish, add the tuna, and turn to coat completely.

4. Place in the grill pan and grill for 1 to 2 minutes per side, or until browned or cooked to desired doneness. Thinly slice each piece of tuna and serve.

*To make this a gluten-free recipe, use gluten-free soy sauce or pure tamari, pure wasabi paste, and nonstick cooking spray with no flour added.

Exchanges
1/2 Carbohydrate
4 Lean Meat

Calories	243
Calories from Fat	93
Total Fat	10 g
Saturated Fat	2.2 g
Cholesterol	42 mg
Sodium	1013 mg
Total Carbohydrate	7 g
Dietary Fiber	1 g
Sugars	5 g
Protein	30 g

"The term 'Ahi' is really just the Hawaiian name for yellowfin tuna. Nowadays we can find it at most major supermarkets because of its popularity—and it's a perfect anytime meal since it cooks up in a flash!"

Tomato-Basil Salmon

Serving Size: 1 fillet; Total Servings: 4

1 tablespoon olive oil

1 medium onion, chopped

2 garlic cloves, minced

1 large tomato, chopped

1/4 teaspoon salt

1/4 teaspoon black pepper

4 salmon fillets (4 ounces each)

1/2 cup dry white wine

1/4 cup low-sodium chicken broth*

1/4 cup chopped fresh basil

1 tablespoon tomato paste

1 In a large skillet, heat the oil over medium heat. Add the onion and garlic; sauté for 3 to 4 minutes or until tender. Stir in the tomato, salt, and pepper; cover, reduce the heat to low, and simmer for 5 minutes.

2 Add the salmon to the skillet then add the wine and chicken broth. Cover and cook for 7 minutes.

3 Uncover the skillet, stir in the basil and tomato paste, and simmer for 4 to 5 minutes, or until the sauce is reduced and the salmon flakes easily with a fork. Serve the salmon topped with sauce.

*To make this a gluten-free recipe, use gluten-free chicken broth.

Exchanges
1 Vegetable
4 Lean Meat
1/2 Fat

Calories 261
  Calories from Fat . . 120
Total Fat . . . . 13 g
  Saturated Fat . . . . . . 2.2 g
Cholesterol . . . . 77 mg
Sodium . . . . 218 mg
Total Carbohydrate . . . . 7 g
  Dietary Fiber . . . . 1 g
  Sugars . . . . 3 g
Protein . . . . 25 g

"I've said it before, but it's important enough to mention again that omega-3 fatty acids are considered 'good fats' and are essential to good health. Salmon is high in this type of fat, which studies have shown can lower blood pressure and cholesterol. Since our bodies can't make omega-3 fatty acids, be sure to include foods that contain it in your meal plan. Your heart will thank you for it!"

Cinnamon-Spiced Snapper

Serving Size: 1 fillet; Total Servings: 6

Nonstick cooking spray*

1 medium onion, cut in half and sliced

1 can (14-1/2 ounces) stewed tomatoes, undrained, broken up

1/3 cup dry white wine

3 tablespoons fresh lemon juice

1 teaspoon ground cumin*

1/8 teaspoon ground cinnamon*

6 red snapper fillets (4 ounces each)

1 Coat a large skillet with nonstick cooking spray.

2 Heat the skillet over medium-high heat. Add the onion; cook for 3 to 4 minutes, or until tender, stirring constantly.

3 Add the tomatoes, wine, lemon juice, cumin, and cinnamon; cook for 5 to 7 minutes, or until the sauce is slightly thickened.

4 Add the snapper to the skillet. Spoon the sauce over the top, cover, and cook over medium heat for 8 to 10 minutes, or until the fish flakes easily with a fork. Serve the fish topped with sauce.

*To make this a gluten-free recipe, use nonstick cooking spray with no flour added, and seasonings with no added starch from a gluten-containing source.

Exchanges
2 Vegetable
3 Very Lean Meat

Calories 148
 Calories from Fat . . . 16
Total Fat . . . . 2 g
 Saturated Fat . . . . . . 0.3 g
Cholesterol . . . . 41 mg
Sodium . . . . 227 mg
Total Carbohydrate . . . . 8 g
 Dietary Fiber . . . . 1 g
 Sugars . . . . 3 g
Protein . . . . 24 g

Preparation Tip

To help speed up your preparation, have your fish cleaned and prepared when you buy it. The fish sellers can remove the skin, portion out your fish, and even remove the bones in many cases. It's like having an extra pair of hands in the kitchen!

Citrus Splash Halibut

Serving Size: 1 piece; Total Servings: 4

Nonstick cooking spray*

1 medium onion, chopped

1 garlic clove, minced

4 halibut steaks or fillets
(4 ounces each)

1/2 teaspoon salt

1/4 teaspoon lemon-pepper
seasoning*

1/2 cup fresh orange juice

1 tablespoon fresh lemon juice

2 tablespoons minced fresh
parsley

1 Coat a large skillet with nonstick
cooking spray.

2 Preheat the skillet over medium
heat; sauté the onion and garlic
until tender.

3 Add the halibut to the skillet;
season with salt and lemon-
pepper then drizzle with orange
juice and lemon juice and
sprinkle with parsley.

4 Cover and cook over medium-
low heat for 10 to 12 minutes, or
until the fish flakes easily with a
fork.

*To make this a gluten-free recipe, use
nonstick cooking spray with no flour
added, and seasoning with no added
starch from a gluten-containing source.

Exchanges
2 Vegetable
3 Very Lean Meat

Calories 156
Calories from Fat . . . 24
Total Fat . . . . 3 g
Saturated Fat . . . . . . 0.4 g
Cholesterol . . . . 36 mg
Sodium . . . . 378 mg
Total Carbohydrate . . . . 8 g
Dietary Fiber . . . . 1 g
Sugars . . . . 5 g
Protein . . . . 24 g

*"An easy way to add
flavor to all your dishes,
but especially fish, is to
add citrus to the other
seasonings—grated
lemon, lime, or orange zest (the
outermost skin) or fresh juice."*

Sea Bass Florentine

Serving Size: 1 fillet; Total Servings: 4

Nonstick cooking spray*

1 cup matchstick-cut carrots, divided

4 sea bass fillets (4 ounces each), rinsed and patted dry

1 lemon, cut in half

1/2 teaspoon salt

1/4 teaspoon black pepper

1 package (10 ounces) fresh spinach, trimmed

1 can (5-1/2 ounces) low-sodium vegetable juice

1 Preheat the oven to 375°F. Coat a 9" x 13" baking dish with non-stick cooking spray.

2 Spread half the carrots evenly over the bottom of the baking dish. Place the fish fillets over the carrots.

3 Squeeze one lemon half over the fish; season with salt and pepper.

4 Distribute the spinach over the fish. Squeeze the remaining lemon half over the spinach; top with the remaining carrots. Pour the vegetable juice over the top; cover the dish tightly with aluminum foil.

5 Bake for 30 to 35 minutes, or until the fish flakes easily with a fork. Serve the fish with the spinach and carrots.

*To make this a gluten-free recipe, use nonstick cooking spray with no flour added.

Exchanges
2 Vegetable
3 Very Lean Meat

Calories	150
Calories from Fat	24
Total Fat	3 g
Saturated Fat	0.1 g
Cholesterol	47 mg
Sodium	474 mg
Total Carbohydrate	9 g
Dietary Fiber	3 g
Sugars	3 g
Protein	23 g

"Why wait for a special occasion to serve up this fancy meal—especially when it's this easy to make?! If you have about a half-hour, you'll have time to throw it together and gather the whole family around the table, even on a busy weeknight!"

Quick Cilantro Pesto Fillets

Serving Size: 1 fillet; Total Servings: 4

Nonstick cooking spray*

1 cup packed cilantro leaves

3 garlic cloves

2 tablespoons fresh lemon juice

1/4 teaspoon salt

1/8 teaspoon ground red pepper*

2 tablespoons olive oil

4 tilapia fillets (4 ounces each)

1 Preheat the oven to 400°F. Coat a 9" x 13" baking dish with non-stick cooking spray.

2 In a food processor or blender, process the cilantro, garlic, lemon juice, salt, and ground red pepper until the cilantro is well chopped, scraping down the sides as needed. Slowly add the oil and process until well blended.

3 Place the tilapia fillets in the baking dish and spread the cilantro pesto evenly over it.

4 Bake for 10 to 12 minutes, or until the fish flakes easily with a fork.

*To make this a gluten-free recipe, use nonstick cooking spray with no flour added, and seasoning with no added starch from a gluten-containing source.

Exchanges
3 Very Lean Meat
1-1/2 Fat

Calories 177
    Calories from Fat . . . 84
Total Fat . . . . 9 g
    Saturated Fat . . . . . . 1.9 g
Cholesterol . . . . 76 mg
Sodium . . . . 181 mg
Total Carbohydrate . . . . 1 g
    Dietary Fiber . . . . 0 g
    Sugars . . . . 1 g
Protein . . . . 23 g

"Pesto is one of those sauces that teams with practically anything. Use it to dress up your regular chicken and fish dishes and even give new life to ordinary sandwiches!"

Asian Trout Bundles

Serving Size: 1 fillet; Total Servings: 4

4 trout fillets (4 ounces each)

1 large red bell pepper, cut into strips

4 scallions, thinly sliced

2 tablespoons light soy sauce*

2 tablespoons balsamic vinegar

2 teaspoons sesame oil

1/2 teaspoon ground ginger*

4 teaspoons sesame seeds

---

*To make this a gluten-free recipe, use gluten-free soy sauce or pure tamari and seasoning with no added starch from a gluten-containing source.

1 Preheat the oven to 425°F.

2 Tear and lay out four 12" x 14" aluminum foil sheets; place 1 trout fillet on each piece of foil.

3 In a medium bowl, combine the bell pepper, scallions, soy sauce, balsamic vinegar, sesame oil, and ginger. Pour the mixture over the fish fillets, dividing it evenly; sprinkle each fillet with 1 teaspoon sesame seeds.

4 Fold the foil over the fish and crimp to seal tightly. Arrange the packets on a baking sheet.

5 Bake for 10 to 12 minutes, or until the fish flakes easily with a fork. Serve in the packets or open the packets and serve (see Tip).

Exchanges

1 Vegetable
3 Lean Meat
1/2 Fat

Calories 227
   Calories from Fat . . . 92
Total Fat . . . . 10 g
   Saturated Fat . . . . . . 2.4 g
Cholesterol . . . . 69 mg
Sodium . . . . 325 mg
Total Carbohydrate . . . . 7 g
   Dietary Fiber . . . . 2 g
   Sugars . . . . 4 g
Protein . . . . 26 g

Serving Tip

For a unique presentation, leave the packets sealed until you're ready to serve then open them at the table. Just be sure to keep your face and hands away as you open the packets, because steam will escape . . . and it's hot!

Fast 'n' Fiery Grilled Catfish

Serving Size: 1 fillet; Total Servings: 4

Nonstick cooking spray*

1 tablespoon chopped fresh basil

1 teaspoon crushed red pepper*

1 teaspoon garlic powder*

1/2 teaspoon salt

1/2 teaspoon black pepper

4 farm-raised catfish fillets (about 6 ounces each)

2 tablespoons canola oil

1 Preheat the grill to medium-high heat. Coat a hinged grill basket with nonstick cooking spray (see Tip).

2 In a small bowl, combine the basil, crushed red pepper, garlic powder, salt, and black pepper; mix well.

3 Rinse the fish with cold water and pat dry with a paper towel. Rub the oil over both sides of the fish then rub both sides with the seasoning mixture, coating evenly.

4 Place the fish in the grill basket and grill for 7 to 9 minutes, or until cooked through and firm to the touch, turning the basket over once during cooking.

---

*To make this a gluten-free recipe, use nonstick cooking spray with no flour added, and seasonings with no added starch from a gluten-containing source.

Exchanges
4 Lean Meat
1 Fat

Calories 274
  Calories from Fat . . 161
Total Fat . . . . 18 g
  Saturated Fat . . . . . . 3.0 g
Cholesterol . . . . 88 mg
Sodium . . . . 402 mg
Total Carbohydrate . . . . 1 g
  Dietary Fiber . . . . 0 g
  Sugars . . . . 0 g
Protein . . . . 26 g

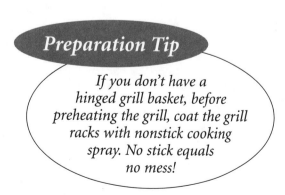

Preparation Tip

If you don't have a hinged grill basket, before preheating the grill, coat the grill racks with nonstick cooking spray. No stick equals no mess!

Meatless Main Dishes

Veggie Hash in a Dash

Serving Size: 1 cup; Total Servings: 6

2 tablespoons olive oil

2 medium onions, chopped

2 bell peppers (1 red and
1 yellow), chopped

2 garlic cloves, minced

1 pound frozen cubed potatoes,
thawed (4 cups)

1/2 pound fresh mushrooms,
quartered

1 box (10 ounces) frozen
asparagus cuts, thawed

1/2 teaspoon salt

1/4 teaspoon black pepper

1 In a large skillet, heat the oil over medium-high heat. Add the onions, bell peppers, and garlic; sauté for 5 minutes, or until the vegetables are tender.

2 Add the potatoes and mushrooms; cook for 10 to 15 minutes, or until the potatoes are lightly browned, stirring frequently.

3 Add the asparagus, salt, and black pepper; cook until heated through. Serve immediately.

Thumbs-up for gluten-free meal plans!

Exchanges

1 Starch
2 Vegetable
1 Fat

Calories 166
  Calories from Fat . . . 50
Total Fat . . . . 6 g
  Saturated Fat . . . . . . 0.8 g
Cholesterol . . . . 0 mg
Sodium . . . . 247 mg
Total Carbohydrate . . . 28 g
  Dietary Fiber . . . . 4 g
  Sugar . . . . 6 g
Protein . . . . 5 g

"Who said you can't enjoy breakfast for dinner? I love to make this anytime eye-opener with whatever veggies I have on hand in my fridge or freezer. That's what makes it so quick to throw together, and it sure beats the everyday hash brown blues!"

Anytime Fried Rice

2 tablespoons sesame oil

3 cups cold cooked white rice, rinsed*

2 cups frozen peas and carrots, thawed

6 scallions, thinly sliced

3 tablespoons light soy sauce*

1/4 cup vegetable broth* (see Options)

1/4 teaspoon black pepper

1 In a large skillet or wok, heat the oil over medium-high heat. Add the rice; stir-fry for 8 to 10 minutes.

2 Add the peas and carrots and the scallions; stir-fry for 1 minute.

3 Add the soy sauce, vegetable broth, and pepper; mix well. Reduce the heat to medium-low and cook, stirring constantly, for 2 to 3 minutes, or until thoroughly mixed and heated through.

*To make this a gluten-free recipe, use rice that has not been enriched, gluten-free soy sauce or pure tamari, and gluten-free vegetable broth.

Exchanges
3 Starch
1 Fat

Calories 277
    Calories from Fat . . . 67
Total Fat . . . . 7 g
    Saturated Fat . . . . . . 1.1 g
Cholesterol . . . . 0 mg
Sodium . . . . 551 mg
Total Carbohydrate . . . 43 g
    Dietary Fiber . . . . 3 g
    Sugar . . . . 5 g
Protein . . . . 7 g

Options

Want to give your fried rice an even bigger flavor boost? Simply substitute low-sodium chicken broth for the vegetable broth and serve it up as-is or alongside your favorite Asian meal.

Mushroom and Zucchini Risotto

Serving Size: 1 cup; Total Servings: 6

Nonstick cooking spray*

2 medium onions, chopped

1/2 pound fresh mushrooms, sliced

2 teaspoons minced garlic

2 cups long- or whole-grain rice*

1 medium zucchini, coarsely shredded

1 can (14 ounces) ready-to-use vegetable broth*

3 cups water

2 teaspoons dried Italian seasoning*

1/2 teaspoon salt

1/4 teaspoon black pepper

1/2 cup grated real Parmesan cheese

1 Coat a large saucepan with nonstick cooking spray.

2 Add the onions, mushrooms, and garlic; sauté over medium-high heat for 5 minutes, or until the onions are tender.

3 Add the rice and zucchini and cook for 3 to 5 minutes, or until the rice begins to brown.

4 Meanwhile, in a medium saucepan, combine vegetable broth, water, Italian seasoning, salt, and pepper; bring to a boil over medium-high heat. Add to the rice mixture, cover, and simmer over low heat for 18 to 20 minutes.

5 Add the Parmesan cheese; stir for 1 to 2 minutes, until creamy and well combined and all the liquid is absorbed. Serve immediately.

*To make this a gluten-free recipe, use nonstick cooking spray with no flour added, rice that has not been enriched, gluten-free vegetable broth, and seasoning with no added starch from a gluten-containing source.

Exchanges
3-1/2 Starch
2 Vegetable

Calories 324
  Calories from Fat . . . 30
Total Fat . . . . 3 g
  Saturated Fat . . . . . . 1.5 g
Cholesterol . . . . 7 mg
Sodium . . . . 524 mg
Total Carbohydrate . . . 63 g
  Dietary Fiber . . . . 2 g
  Sugar . . . . 5 g
Protein . . . . 10 g

Did You Know . . .

that risotto is a healthy alternative to traditional pastas? It's perfect for busy weeknight suppers. Just be sure to watch your carbohydrate total!

Five-Minute Tex-Mex Couscous

Serving Size: 1-1/3 cups; Total Servings: 6

1 package (10 ounces) couscous*

1 can (15-1/2 ounces) black beans, drained and rinsed

1 can (15-1/2 ounces) corn, drained and rinsed

2 tomatoes, diced

2 tablespoons fresh minced cilantro

1 teaspoon ground cumin*

1/2 teaspoon salt

1 Cook the couscous according to the package directions.

2 In a bowl, combine the remaining ingredients; mix well. Add the couscous; mix until well combined. Serve at room temperature, or cover and refrigerate for serving cold.

*To make this a gluten-free recipe, use quinoa instead of couscous and use seasoning with no added starch from a gluten-containing source.

Exchanges

3-1/2 Starch

Calories 260
  Calories from Fat . . . 10
Total Fat . . . . 1 g
  Saturated Fat . . . . . . 0.2 g
Cholesterol . . . . 0 mg
Sodium . . . . 353 mg
Total Carbohydrate . . . 53 g
  Dietary Fiber . . . . 7 g
  Sugar . . . . 3 g
Protein . . . . 11 g

Did You Know . . .

that couscous is coarsely ground semolina pasta, popular in North African and Middle Eastern cooking? This recipe brings two cultures together for a side dish that blends the flavors of the American Southwest with the quick-cooking ease of a Mediterranean favorite!

Veggie Frittata

Serving Size: 1 wedge; Total Servings: 4

Nonstick cooking spray*

1 cup cut fresh asparagus

1 cup chopped fresh mushrooms

1/2 cup chopped broccoli florets

2 scallions, thinly sliced

1/2 red bell pepper, chopped

1 garlic clove, crushed

1/8 teaspoon crushed red pepper* (optional)

1/2 teaspoon salt

3 whole eggs

3 egg whites

1/4 cup nonfat milk

---

*To make this a gluten-free recipe, use nonstick cooking spray with no flour added and, if using crushed red pepper, use a brand with no added starch from a gluten-containing source.

Exchanges
1 Vegetable
1 Medium-Fat Meat

Calories 99
 Calories from Fat . . . 37
Total Fat . . . . 4 g
 Saturated Fat . . . . . . 1.2 g
Cholesterol . . . . 159 mg
Sodium . . . . 401 mg
Total Carbohydrate . . . . 6 g
 Dietary Fiber . . . . 2 g
 Sugar . . . . 4 g
Protein . . . . 10 g

1 Coat a 10-inch nonstick skillet with nonstick cooking spray; heat over medium-high heat.

2 Add the asparagus, mushrooms, broccoli, scallions, bell pepper, garlic, crushed red pepper, if desired, and salt. Cook for 2 to 3 minutes, or until the vegetables are tender, stirring occasionally.

3 Meanwhile, in a medium bowl, whisk together the whole eggs, egg whites, and milk. Reduce the heat of the skillet to medium-low and add the egg mixture.

4 As the mixture begins to set, push the cooked edges slightly toward the center, allowing the liquid to run to the edges of the skillet. Reduce the heat to low, cover, and cook for 8 to 9 minutes, or until the eggs are set.

5 Slide the frittata onto a serving platter. Cut into 4 wedges and serve immediately.

"Say goodbye to boring omelets and hello to frittatas! So what's the difference? A frittata is basically an open-faced omelet with all the ingredients mixed right in with the eggs and cooked slowly over a low heat. Besides being packed with protein, this frittata sure makes a colorful presentation!"

Zesty Lasagna Roll-Ups

Serving Size: 1 roll-up; Total Servings: 8

8 lasagna noodles*

Nonstick cooking spray*

1 cup shredded reduced-fat
Cheddar cheese, divided

1 container (15 ounces) fat-free
ricotta cheese

1 can (4 ounces) chopped green
chilies, drained

1/2 teaspoon chili powder*

1/8 teaspoon salt

1 can (15-1/2 ounces) pinto
beans, drained and rinsed

1 cup salsa

---

*To make this a gluten-free recipe, use a
gluten-free noodle substitute, nonstick
cooking spray with no flour added, and
seasoning with no added starch from a
gluten-containing source.

1 Cook the lasagna noodles
according to the package directions; drain and let cool.

2 Preheat the oven to 350°F. Coat
a 7" x 11" baking dish with nonstick cooking spray.

3 In a large bowl, combine 1/2 cup
Cheddar cheese, the ricotta
cheese, green chilies, chili powder, and salt; mix well. Add the
pinto beans, mixing gently.

4 Lay the lasagna noodles on a flat
surface, spread the cheese mixture evenly over the noodles then
roll them up jellyroll-style.

5 Place the lasagna rolls seam-side
down in the baking dish. Spoon
the salsa over the top and sprinkle with the remaining 1/2 cup
Cheddar cheese.

6 Bake for 20 to 25 minutes, or
until heated through.

Exchanges
2 Starch
1 Lean Meat

Calories 226	
Calories from Fat . . . 33	
Total Fat . . . . 4 g	
Saturated Fat . . . . . . 1.8 g	
Cholesterol . . . . 27 mg	
Sodium . . . . 481 mg	
Total Carbohydrate . . . 32 g	
Dietary Fiber . . . . 5 g	
Sugar . . . . 5 g	
Protein . . . . 17 g	

*"What makes these indi-
vidual lasagna roll-ups
so unique is that you
can tailor the ingredients
to whatever each person
likes! If you're cooking for someone
who doesn't like spicy food, leave
out the green chilies and chili
powder, roll some roll-ups, and
then add an adjusted amount of
chilies and chili powder to the rest
of the mixture and roll away. It's
that easy!"*

Cheesy Spinach Quiche

Serving Size: 1 slice; Total Servings: 8

3/4 cup egg substitute

1 cup fat-free milk

1 cup shredded fat-free real
Cheddar cheese

1 cup shredded reduced-fat real
Swiss cheese

1 package (10 ounces) frozen
chopped spinach, thawed (see
Note)

1 teaspoon onion powder*

1/4 teaspoon ground nutmeg*

1/2 teaspoon salt

1/4 teaspoon black pepper

1 nine-inch ready-to-bake deep-
dish reduced-fat pie crust*
(optional)

Nonstick cooking spray*

8 cups broccoli florets

See photo insert following page 36.

Exchanges

2 Vegetable
2 Very Lean Meat

Calories 108
  Calories from Fat . . . 20
Total Fat . . . . 2 g
  Saturated Fat . . . . . . 1.1 g
Cholesterol . . . . 7 mg
Sodium . . . . 407 mg
Total Carbohydrate . . . . 8 g
  Dietary Fiber . . . . 3 g
  Sugar . . . . 4 g
Protein . . . . 15 g

1 Preheat the oven to 350°F.

2 In a medium bowl, beat the egg
substitute and milk until well
combined. Add the Cheddar
cheese, Swiss cheese, spinach,
onion powder, nutmeg, salt, and
pepper; mix well then pour into
the pie crust, if desired, or a
9-inch pie plate coated with
nonstick cooking spray.

3 Bake for 40 to 45 minutes, or
until firm. Let sit for 5 minutes.

4 Meanwhile, steam the broccoli
florets for 3 to 4 minutes, or until
crisp-tender.

5 Slice quiche and serve with
broccoli florets.

*To make this a gluten-free recipe, use
seasonings with no added starch from a
gluten-containing source, nonstick
cooking spray with no flour added, and
a gluten-free pie crust, if using one.

*"What was once a brunch
staple has fast become a
dinnertime treat! And
because spinach is filled
with vitamins, minerals,
and fiber, it's a great bonus in this
easy, cheesy dish! Plus, it's up to
you to include the crust or not—
this works just as well crustless."*

Grilled Pita Pizzas

Serving Size: 1 pizza; Total Servings: 4

4 six-inch whole wheat pita breads*

1/2 cup light spaghetti sauce*

1 cup broccoli florets

1/2 red bell pepper, cut into thin strips

1/2 green bell pepper, cut into thin strips

2 tablespoons sliced black olives

1/2 cup shredded part-skim real mozzarella cheese

See photo insert following page 84.

1 Preheat the grill to medium heat.

2 Spread each pita bread evenly with sauce then top with broccoli, pepper strips, olives, and shredded cheese.

3 Place pizzas on grill rack; close the cover and cook for 8 to 10 minutes, or until heated through and the cheese is melted. Serve immediately.

*To make this a gluten-free recipe, use gluten-free individual pizza crusts and gluten-free spaghetti sauce.

Exchanges
2 Starch
1 Vegetable
1/2 Fat

Calories 207
Calories from Fat . . . 40
Total Fat . . . . 4 g
Saturated Fat . . . . . . 1.6 g
Cholesterol . . . . 8 mg
Sodium . . . . 393 mg
Total Carbohydrate . . . 36 g
Dietary Fiber . . . . 4 g
Sugar . . . . 5 g
Protein . . . . 10 g

"This is such a great party food! It's fun to put out different vegetables and seasonings like basil, oregano, Italian seasoning, and garlic, and let your guests design their own creations. If you prefer to bake these pizzas instead of grilling them, put them in a pre-heated 400°F. oven for 10 to 12 minutes, or until the pitas are crisp and the cheese is melted."

Side Dishes

Honey Stir-Fried Vegetables

Serving Size: 1/2 cup; Total Servings: 12

6 garlic cloves, minced

1/4 cup honey

1 tablespoon light soy sauce*

1 tablespoon cornstarch

1 teaspoon sesame seeds

1/2 cup vegetable broth*

1 pound fresh wax beans, trimmed

1/3 pound fresh snow peas, trimmed

1 large red bell pepper, cut into 1/4-inch strips

1 In a small bowl, combine the garlic, honey, soy sauce, and cornstarch; mix well and set aside.

2 In a large skillet or wok, toast the sesame seeds over medium heat for 2 to 3 minutes, until golden, stirring frequently.

3 Add the vegetable broth and wax beans to the skillet; cook for 5 minutes, stirring occasionally.

4 Add the snow peas and bell pepper; cook for 2 minutes, stirring constantly. Add the honey mixture; mix well. Cook for 2 minutes, or until the sauce thickens, stirring occasionally. Serve immediately.

*To make this a gluten-free recipe, use gluten-free soy sauce or pure tamari and gluten-free vegetable broth.

Exchanges
1/2 Carbohydrate

Calories 49
    Calories from Fat 3
Total Fat . . . . 0 g
    Saturated Fat . . . . . . 0.1 g
Cholesterol . . . . 0 mg
Sodium . . . . 90 mg
Total Carbohydrate . . . 11 g
    Dietary Fiber . . . . 2 g
    Sugars . . . . 8 g
Protein . . . . 1 g

"Serve your honey this namesake any night of the week and watch the sparks fly! The sweet honey paired with the full-bodied soy sauce makes the best-tasting reason to avoid calling for take-out."

Mixed-Up Roasted Vegetables

Serving Size: 1/2 cup; Total Servings: 8

Nonstick cooking spray*

2 medium-sized yellow squash, cut into 1/2-inch slices

2 medium-sized zucchini, cut into 1/2-inch slices

1 medium-sized onion, quartered

2 medium-sized bell peppers (1 red, 1 green), cut into 1/2-inch chunks

1 tablespoon canola oil

1/2 teaspoon garlic powder*

1/2 teaspoon salt

1/2 teaspoon black pepper

1 Preheat the oven to 450°F. Coat a large rimmed baking sheet with nonstick cooking spray.

2 In a large bowl, combine all the vegetables; toss to mix.

3 In a small bowl, combine the remaining ingredients; mix well. Drizzle over the vegetable mixture; toss until well coated.

4 Lay out the vegetables in a single layer on the baking sheet. Roast for 28 to 30 minutes, or until the vegetables are tender, turning halfway through cooking. Serve.

---

*To make this a gluten-free recipe, use nonstick cooking spray with no flour added, and seasoning with no added starch from a gluten-containing source.

Exchanges
2 Vegetable

Calories 50
   Calories from Fat . . . 18
Total Fat . . . . 2 g
   Saturated Fat . . . . . . 0.2 g
Cholesterol . . . . 0 mg
Sodium . . . . 153 mg
Total Carbohydrate . . . . 8 g
   Dietary Fiber . . . . 2 g
   Sugars . . . . 4 g
Protein . . . . 2 g

"I just love roasted vegetables! They mix and cook up in a flash, and they add terrific color and life to any meal. Best of all, you can pretty much use any combination of fresh vegetables that you have on hand for a sure way to avoid the dinnertime rut!"

Italian Roasted Tomatoes

Serving Size: 1 tomato half; Total Servings: 8

Nonstick cooking spray*

4 medium-sized ripe tomatoes

2 tablespoons olive oil

2 teaspoons minced garlic

1/2 teaspoon onion powder*

1/4 teaspoon dried oregano*

1/4 teaspoon salt

1/4 teaspoon black pepper

2 tablespoons grated real Parmesan cheese

2 tablespoons chopped fresh basil

1 Preheat the oven to 450°F. Coat a 9" x 13" baking dish with non-stick cooking spray.

2 Core the tomatoes and cut in half horizontally; place in the baking dish cut-side up.

3 In a small bowl, combine the oil, garlic, onion powder, oregano, salt, and pepper; mix well. Evenly brush the cut sides of the tomatoes with the mixture.

4 Sprinkle the tops evenly with Parmesan cheese. Bake for 20 to 22 minutes, or until the tomatoes are soft and the tops are browned. Sprinkle with basil and serve.

*To make this a gluten-free recipe, use nonstick cooking spray with no flour added, and seasonings with no added starch from a gluten-containing source.

Exchanges
1 Vegetable
1/2 Fat

Calories 49
  Calories from Fat . . . 36
Total Fat . . . . 4 g
  Saturated Fat . . . . . . 0.7 g
Cholesterol . . . . 1 mg
Sodium . . . . 87 mg
Total Carbohydrate . . . . 3 g
  Dietary Fiber . . . . 1 g
  Sugars . . . . 2 g
Protein . . . . 1 g

"Don't save all your tomatoes for the salad! Keep some aside for this fresh-as-can-be side dish. Roasting tomatoes is a super way to bring out their sweet juices and makes for an easy, low-carb go-along."

Baked Balsamic Asparagus

Serving Size: 1/6 recipe; Total Servings: 6

1 pound fresh asparagus, trimmed

2 tablespoons olive oil

2 tablespoons balsamic vinegar

1/4 teaspoon salt

1/4 teaspoon black pepper

1 Preheat the oven to 350°F. Cut a sheet of aluminum foil 18 inches long.

2 Place the asparagus on the foil; drizzle with oil and vinegar then sprinkle with salt and pepper. Seal the foil packet and place it on a baking sheet.

3 Bake for 12 to 15 minutes, or until the asparagus is tender. Open the packet carefully and serve.

Thumbs-up for gluten-free meal plans!

Exchanges
1 Vegetable
1 Fat

Calories 52
  Calories from Fat . . . 42
Total Fat . . . . 5 g
  Saturated Fat . . . . . . 0.6 g
Cholesterol . . . . 0 mg
Sodium . . . . 101 mg
Total Carbohydrate . . . . 3 g
  Dietary Fiber . . . . 1 g
  Sugars . . . . 1 g
Protein . . . . 1 g

"The woody flavor of balsamic vinegar guarantees a great salad dressing. But I like to use balsamic vinegar in everything from mixed salads and marinades to grilled vegetables and so much more. It adds robust flavor to our dishes . . . without any guilt."

Too-Easy Tarragon Asparagus

Serving Size: 1/6 recipe; Total Servings: 6

1 pound fresh asparagus, trimmed

1 tablespoon butter, cut up

1 tablespoon fresh lemon juice

1 tablespoon dried tarragon*

1 Preheat the oven to 350°F.

2 Place the asparagus in a shallow baking dish. Dot with butter, drizzle with lemon juice, and sprinkle with tarragon. Cover with aluminum foil.

3 Bake for 12 to 15 minutes, or until the asparagus is tender. Serve immediately.

---

*To make this a gluten-free recipe, use seasoning with no added starch from a gluten-containing source.

Exchanges
1 Vegetable

Calories 27
   Calories from Fat . . . 19
Total Fat . . . . 2 g
   Saturated Fat . . . . . . 1.2 g
Cholesterol . . . . 5 mg
Sodium . . . . 18 mg
Total Carbohydrate . . . . 2 g
   Dietary Fiber . . . . 1 g
   Sugars . . . . 1 g
Protein . . . . 1 g

"Asparagus is one of my favorite vegetables, and this is one of my favorite ways to have it. Mr. Food even taught me how to choose asparagus: Look for firm, bright green stalks with tight tips. Store your asparagus in a plastic bag in the refrigerator so that it stays fresh and green until you're ready to enjoy it."

Green Beans Italiano

Serving Size: 1/2 cup; Total Servings: 10

1 pound green beans, trimmed

1 tablespoon olive oil

2 garlic cloves, minced

1/8 teaspoon black pepper

1/4 cup shredded real Parmesan cheese

1 Bring a soup pot of water to a boil over high heat. Add the green beans; blanch for 5 to 6 minutes.

2 Meanwhile, in a large skillet, heat the oil over medium heat. Add the garlic; sauté until golden.

3 Add the green beans and black pepper; sauté for 3 minutes, or until crisp-tender. Sprinkle with Parmesan cheese and serve.

Thumbs-up for gluten-free meal plans!

Exchanges

1 Vegetable

Calories 36
  Calories from Fat . . . 20
Total Fat . . . . 2 g
  Saturated Fat . . . . . . 0.6 g
Cholesterol . . . . 2 mg
Sodium . . . . 19 mg
Total Carbohydrate . . . . 3 g
  Dietary Fiber . . . . 1 g
  Sugars . . . . 1 g
Protein . . . . 2 g

"Sure, you could buy canned green beans ready to heat and eat, but there's nothing more delicious than fresh. They're so versatile—they work well with whatever flavors you team them with, so try tossing up this terrific combination today."

Crunchy Baked Green Beans

Serving Size: 1/2 cup; Total Servings: 8

Nonstick cooking spray*

1 package (16 ounces) frozen green beans, thawed

1 can (10-3/4 ounces) reduced-fat condensed cream of mushroom soup*

1 can (8 ounces) sliced water chestnuts, drained

1/4 teaspoon onion powder*

1/4 teaspoon black pepper

1 Preheat the oven to 350°F. Coat a 7" x 11" baking dish with non-stick cooking spray.

2 Combine all the ingredients in a large bowl; mix well. Spoon the mixture into the baking dish.

3 Bake for 35 to 40 minutes, or until the beans are tender and heated through. Serve immediately.

---

*To make this a gluten-free recipe, use nonstick cooking spray with no flour added, gluten-free soup, and seasoning with no added starch from a gluten-containing source.

Exchanges
1 Vegetable

Calories 42
  Calories from Fat 8
Total Fat . . . . 1 g
  Saturated Fat . . . . . . 0.3 g
Cholesterol . . . . 1 mg
Sodium . . . . 276 mg
Total Carbohydrate . . . . 8 g
  Dietary Fiber . . . . 3 g
  Sugars . . . . 2 g
Protein . . . . 1 g

"This is one of my specialties that my family asks for pretty regularly. Sometimes we even like to sprinkle on a bit of grated real Parmesan cheese as a nice flavor accent."

Steamin' Greens

Serving Size: 1/2 cup; Total Servings: 8

1/4 cup olive oil

8 cups Steamin' Greens (see Note)

1/3 cup low-sodium chicken broth*

4 garlic cloves, minced

1/8 teaspoon salt

1/4 teaspoon black pepper

1 In a large skillet, heat the oil over medium-high heat. Add the Steamin' Greens; sauté for 2 minutes.

2 Stir in the remaining ingredients, cover, and cook for 8 to 10 minutes, or until the Steamin' Greens are tender.

*To make this a gluten-free recipe, use gluten-free chicken broth.

Exchanges
1 Vegetable
1-1/2 Fat

Calories 83
Calories from Fat . . . 64
Total Fat . . . . 7 g
Saturated Fat . . . . . . 1.0 g
Cholesterol . . . . 0 mg
Sodium . . . . 96 mg
Total Carbohydrate . . . . 5 g
Dietary Fiber . . . . 1 g
Sugars . . . . 1 g
Protein . . . . 2 g

"Steamin' Greens, a multicolored blend of the vegetables Salad Savoy and Bright Lights, comes as a bite-sized, ready-to-use product. So vibrant that they're often used as a garnish, these versatile vegetables are also packed with nutrition, making them worth adding to as many of our dishes as we can, from soups to main courses and more! Ask your supermarket produce manager for Salad Savoy products or use Swiss chard or kale in this recipe."

Ten-Minute Minty Orzo

Serving Size: 1/2 cup; Total Servings: 10

8 ounces (1-1/2 cups dry) orzo pasta

1 package (10 ounces) frozen peas

1 small onion, chopped

1/2 cup tightly packed fresh mint leaves, chopped

1 tablespoon olive oil

1/4 teaspoon garlic powder

1/4 teaspoon salt

1/4 teaspoon black pepper

1 In a large saucepan, heat 10 cups water to boiling; add the orzo and cook for 5 minutes.

2 Add the frozen peas and the onion; cook for 5 minutes, or until the orzo is done.

3 Drain the orzo then return it to the saucepan and add the remaining ingredients; toss until well combined. Serve immediately.

Exchanges
1-1/2 Starch

Calories 123
  Calories from Fat . . . 16
Total Fat . . . . 2 g
  Saturated Fat . . . . . . 0.2 g
Cholesterol . . . . 0 mg
Sodium . . . . 81 mg
Total Carbohydrate . . . 22 g
  Dietary Fiber . . . . 3 g
  Sugars . . . . 3 g
Protein . . . . 4 g

Did You Know . . .

that orzo is a small, rice-shaped pasta? It has made its way into everything from soups to side dishes and is sure giving rice a run for its money! Keep some orzo in your pantry for those times when you're looking to serve up something a bit out of the ordinary.

Herb-Roasted Potatoes

Serving Size: 1/2 cup; Total Servings: 12

Nonstick cooking spray*

2 teaspoons paprika*

1 teaspoon garlic powder*

1 teaspoon onion powder*

1 teaspoon salt

1/2 teaspoon black pepper

8 medium-sized red-skinned potatoes (about 2-1/2 pounds), washed and cut into 1-inch chunks

1 tablespoon vegetable oil

---

*To make this a gluten-free recipe, use nonstick cooking spray with no flour added, and seasonings with no added starch from a gluten-containing source.

1 Preheat the oven to 400°F. Coat a large rimmed baking sheet with nonstick cooking spray.

2 In a small bowl, combine the paprika, garlic powder, onion powder, salt, and pepper; mix well.

3 In a large bowl, toss the potatoes with oil. Add the spice mixture; toss until the potatoes are well coated. Spread the potatoes in a single layer on the baking sheet.

4 Bake for 45 to 50 minutes, or until fork-tender, turning the potatoes occasionally and coating them with nonstick cooking spray halfway through baking. Serve immediately.

Exchanges
1 Starch

Calories 81
  Calories from Fat . . . 12
Total Fat . . . . 1 g
  Saturated Fat . . . . . . 0.1 g
Cholesterol . . . . 0 mg
Sodium . . . . 200 mg
Total Carbohydrate . . . 16 g
  Dietary Fiber . . . . 2 g
  Sugars . . . . 1 g
Protein . . . . 2 g

Preparation Tip

Want to speed things up? The night before serving these, chunk up the potatoes and place them in a bowl of water; cover them with plastic wrap and store in the refrigerator. This will help keep the potatoes from browning, and they'll be ready and waiting for you to mix up and bake the next day!

Simple Scalloped Potatoes

Serving Size: 1/2 cup; Total Servings: 12

Nonstick cooking spray*

1 can (10-3/4 ounces) reduced-fat condensed cream of mushroom soup*

3/4 cup fat-free milk

1/2 cup reduced-fat sour cream

1 teaspoon onion powder*

1/2 teaspoon salt

1/4 teaspoon white pepper

1 package (30 ounces) frozen shredded potatoes, thawed

1/8 teaspoon paprika*

1 scallion, sliced

---

*To make this a gluten-free recipe, use nonstick cooking spray with no flour added, gluten-free soup, and seasonings with no added starch from a gluten-containing source.

1 Preheat the oven to 400°F. Coat a 2-quart casserole dish with nonstick cooking spray.

2 In a large bowl, combine the soup, milk, sour cream, onion powder, salt, and pepper; mix well. Add the potatoes; toss until evenly coated. Place the coated potatoes in the casserole dish; sprinkle with paprika.

3 Cover the dish and bake for 25 minutes.

4 Uncover and bake for 35 to 40 more minutes, or until heated through and the top is golden. Sprinkle with the scallion and serve immediately.

Exchanges
1 Starch

Calories 94
  Calories from Fat . . . 16
Total Fat . . . . 2 g
  Saturated Fat . . . . . . 0.8 g
Cholesterol . . . . 4 mg
Sodium . . . . 303 mg
Total Carbohydrate . . . 17 g
  Dietary Fiber . . . . 1 g
  Sugars . . . . 2 g
Protein . . . . 3 g

"By using reduced-fat and fat-free dairy products, you can substantially lower the amount of saturated fat in your dishes. So go ahead and enjoy this creamy, homestyle treat! Just remember to control your portions, because this one's sure to have everyone wanting seconds."

Spicy Baked Sweet Potato Fries

Serving Size: 6 fries; Total Servings: 6

Nonstick cooking spray*

1 tablespoon chili powder*

1 teaspoon salt

1/4 teaspoon black pepper

1/4 teaspoon ground red pepper*

3 large sweet potatoes (about 2-1/2 pounds), peeled and cut lengthwise into thin wedges

---

*To make this a gluten-free recipe, use nonstick cooking spray with no flour added, and seasonings with no added starch from a gluten-containing source.

1 Preheat the oven to 425°F. Coat rimmed baking sheets with nonstick cooking spray.

2 In a large resealable plastic storage bag, combine the chili powder, salt, black pepper, and ground red pepper. Add the potato wedges to the bag and shake until completely coated.

3 Spread the potato wedges in a single layer on the baking sheets. Coat the potatoes with nonstick cooking spray.

4 Bake for 22 to 25 minutes, or until golden and tender. Serve immediately.

Exchanges

2 Starch

Calories 137
   Calories from Fat 4
Total Fat . . . . 0 g
   Saturated Fat . . . . . . 0.1 g
Cholesterol . . . . 0 mg
Sodium . . . . 454 mg
Total Carbohydrate . . . 31 g
   Dietary Fiber . . . . 5 g
   Sugars . . . . 13 g
Protein . . . . 3 g

Option

If you're a fan of crispy fries, simply combine the seasonings with 2 beaten egg whites in a shallow dish. Coat the potato wedges with this mixture and bake as above. They'll crisp up in no time!

Maple-Nut Sweet Potato Casserole

Serving Size: 1/2 cup; Total Servings: 8

Nonstick cooking spray*

1 can (29 ounces) sweet
  potatoes, drained

1/2 cup egg substitute

1 teaspoon maple extract*
  (see Option)

1/4 cup chopped pecans

1/4 cup quick-cooking oats*

2 tablespoons light brown sugar

1 tablespoon all-purpose flour*

2 tablespoons light butter,
  softened

1 Preheat the oven to 350°F. Coat an 8-inch square baking dish with nonstick cooking spray.

2 In a large food processor, blend together the sweet potatoes, egg substitute, and maple extract until smooth. Spread the mixture in the baking dish.

3 In a small bowl, combine the remaining ingredients until crumbly. Sprinkle evenly over the top of the potato mixture. Spray the top of the mixture with non-stick cooking spray.

4 Bake for 30 to 35 minutes, or until the top is golden. Serve immediately.

*To make this a gluten-free recipe, use nonstick cooking spray with no flour added, gluten-free extract, Irish oats, and tapioca flour instead of all-purpose flour.

Exchanges
1-1/2 Starch
1 Fat

Calories 156
  Calories from Fat . . . 42
Total Fat . . . . 5 g
  Saturated Fat . . . . . . 1.3 g
Cholesterol . . . . 5 mg
Sodium . . . . 59 mg
Total Carbohydrate . . . 27 g
  Dietary Fiber . . . . 3 g
  Sugars . . . . 15 g
Protein . . . . 4 g

Option

Although the maple flavor is nice in here, if you don't have maple extract on hand, you can always substitute vanilla extract.

Cinnamon-Sugar Apple Rings

Serving Size: 1/2 cup; Total Servings: 10

2 tablespoons light butter

1 tablespoon light brown sugar

3/4 teaspoon ground cinnamon*

3 large apples, peeled, cored, and cut into 1/2-inch-thick rings

1/4 cup chopped walnuts

1 In a large skillet, melt the butter over medium-low heat; add the brown sugar and cinnamon, stirring until blended.

2 Add the apple rings; toss gently to coat. Cover and cook over low heat for 10 to 15 minutes, stirring occasionally.

3 Sprinkle with chopped walnuts and serve.

*To make this a gluten-free recipe, use seasoning with no added starch from a gluten-containing source.

Exchanges
1/2 Fruit
1/2 Fat

Calories 68
  Calories from Fat . . . 30
Total Fat . . . . 3 g
  Saturated Fat . . . . . . 1.0 g
Cholesterol . . . . 4 mg
Sodium . . . . 16 mg
Total Carbohydrate . . . 10 g
  Dietary Fiber . . . . 1 g
  Sugars . . . . 9 g
Protein . . . . 1 g

Did You Know . . .

that the Granny Smith could be called the perfect all-purpose apple? It's available year-round and stands up well to long cooking. You're going to wonder if this is really a side dish, a dessert . . . or both!

Irish Brown Bread

Serving Size: 1 wedge; Total Servings: 16

Nonstick cooking spray

1-1/2 cups whole-wheat flour

1 cup all-purpose flour

1 teaspoon baking soda

1 teaspoon salt

2 tablespoons light butter, cut into small pieces

1 egg

1 cup low-fat buttermilk

1 Preheat the oven to 425°F. Coat a rimmed baking sheet with nonstick cooking spray.

2 In a large bowl, combine the whole-wheat flour, all-purpose flour, baking soda, and salt; mix well.

3 Add the butter then the egg and buttermilk. Using your hands, mix until just combined. Right on the baking sheet, shape the dough into a round loaf about 1 inch high. Make a crisscross cut (an "X") across the top with a floured knife.

4 Bake the bread for 10 minutes. Reduce the oven temperature to 350°F. Bake for 25 to 30 more minutes, or until a toothpick inserted in the center comes out clean. Cool for a bit on a wire rack then cut into wedges and serve warm.

Exchanges
1 Starch

Calories 84
   Calories from Fat . . . 13
Total Fat . . . . 1 g
   Saturated Fat . . . . . . 0.7 g
Cholesterol . . . . 16 mg
Sodium . . . . 255 mg
Total Carbohydrate . . . 15 g
   Dietary Fiber . . . . 2 g
   Sugars . . . . 1 g
Protein . . . . 3 g

"If you can't make it to Ireland anytime soon, bring the taste of Ireland to your table tonight! One of the easiest and quickest breads to bake up, this has become a favorite in my house. I like to slice it up and serve it warm with a little margarine or sugar-free jam on the side."

Spicy Polenta Pancakes

Serving Size: 2 pancakes; Total Servings: 8

1 can (4 ounces) chopped green chilies, drained

3/4 cup low-fat milk

3/4 cup all-purpose flour*

1/2 cup yellow cornmeal

1/2 cup reduced-fat sour cream

1 egg white

1 tablespoon sugar

3/4 teaspoon baking soda

1/2 teaspoon baking powder

1/2 teaspoon ground cumin*

1/4 teaspoon salt

Nonstick cooking spray*

1 In a large bowl, combine all the ingredients except the cooking spray; mix well.

2 Coat a medium skillet or griddle with nonstick cooking spray. Heat over medium heat until a drop of water sizzles on the surface.

3 Pour 2 tablespoons batter per pancake onto the skillet, making 3-inch circles. Cook for 2 to 3 minutes, until bubbles begin to form on the tops and the surface has a dry appearance. Flip the pancakes and cook for 1 to 2 more minutes, or until golden on both sides. Serve immediately.

*To make this a gluten-free recipe, use a gluten-free substitute that works in place of a quantity of all-purpose flour, seasoning with no added starch from a gluten-containing source, and nonstick cooking spray with no flour added.

Exchanges

1-1/2 Starch

Calories	112
Calories from Fat	16
Total Fat	2 g
Saturated Fat	0.9 g
Cholesterol	6 mg
Sodium	273 mg
Total Carbohydrate	20 g
Dietary Fiber	1 g
Sugars	3 g
Protein	4 g

"Elevate these to gourmet level by making them bite-sized and serving them as party hors d'oeuvres, each topped with a drop of salsa and a sprig of fresh cilantro just before serving."

Desserts

Chocolate Biscotti

Serving Size: 1 biscotti; Total Servings: 36

Nonstick cooking spray*

1 cup all-purpose flour*

1/2 cup sugar

1/3 cup unsweetened cocoa

1/2 teaspoon baking soda

1/8 teaspoon salt

2 eggs

1/2 teaspoon vanilla extract

1/2 cup whole blanched almonds

*To make this a gluten-free recipe, use nonstick cooking spray with no flour added, and 1 cup gluten-free flour blend plus 1/4 teaspoon xanthan gum instead of all-purpose flour.

1 Preheat the oven to 350°F. Coat 2 rimmed baking sheets with nonstick cooking spray.

2 In a large bowl, combine all the ingredients except the almonds; mix well with a spoon. Stir in the almonds until well blended. (The dough will be thick and sticky.)

3 Divide the dough into 4 equal parts then shape into 2-inch-high loaves. Place 2 loaves on each baking sheet 2 inches apart.

4 Bake for 15 minutes. Reduce the oven temperature to 325°F.

5 Remove the loaves from the oven and allow to cool for 15 minutes.

6 Cut the loaves into 1/2-inch slices. Lay the slices cut-side down on the baking sheets and bake for 15 more minutes. Turn the slices over and bake for another 15 minutes, or until very crisp.

7 Allow to cool then store in an airtight container.

Exchanges
1/2 Carbohydrate

Calories 41
   Calories from Fat . . . 13
Total Fat . . . . 1 g
   Saturated Fat . . . . . . 0.3 g
Cholesterol . . . . 12 mg
Sodium . . . . 30 mg
Total Carbohydrate . . . . 6 g
   Dietary Fiber . . . . 1 g
   Sugars . . . . 3 g
Protein . . . . 1 g

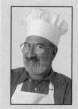

"You've probably seen these crispy cookies in coffee shops and bakeries, but did you know how easy they are to make? They're perfect for dipping in coffee, tea, and milk or enjoying all by themselves. If you want to fancy them up, dip one end in melted chocolate."

Lickety-Split Lemon Oaties

Serving Size: 1 cookie; Total Servings: 30

Nonstick cooking spray

5 tablespoons stick margarine

1/4 cup granulated sugar

1/4 cup packed light brown sugar

2 egg whites

1 tablespoon grated lemon peel

1 cup quick-cooking rolled oats

1/2 cup all-purpose flour

1 Preheat the oven to 350°F. Coat baking sheets with nonstick cooking spray.

2 In a large bowl, beat the margarine, granulated sugar, brown sugar, egg whites, and lemon peel until light and creamy. Add the oats and flour; mix until just blended.

3 Drop the dough by rounded teaspoonfuls 1-1/2 inches apart onto the baking sheets.

4 Bake for 10 to 12 minutes, or until the edges are golden.

5 Remove from the oven and let stand for 3 minutes. Remove the cookies to a wire rack to cool completely.

Exchanges
1/2 Carbohydrate
1/2 Fat

Calories 49
   Calories from Fat ... 19
Total Fat .... 2 g
   Saturated Fat ...... 0.4 g
Cholesterol .... 0 mg
Sodium .... 24 mg
Total Carbohydrate .... 7 g
   Dietary Fiber .... 0 g
   Sugars .... 3 g
Protein .... 1 g

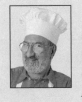

"These are a great change-of-pace cookie, especially when you're looking for something light but packed with flavor."

Orange Walnut Mini Muffins

Serving Size: 1 muffin; Total Servings: 30

Nonstick cooking spray*

1 cup sugar

1/4 cup (1/2 stick) light butter

1 egg

2 teaspoons grated orange peel

1/2 teaspoon vanilla extract*

1/8 teaspoon ground cinnamon*

2 cups whole-wheat flour*

1 teaspoon baking soda

1/2 cup freshly squeezed orange juice

1/2 cup water

1/2 cup chopped walnuts

1 Preheat the oven to 350°F. Coat mini muffin pans with nonstick cooking spray.

2 In a medium bowl, cream the sugar and butter. Add the egg, orange peel, vanilla extract, and cinnamon; mix well.

3 In another medium bowl, combine the flour and baking soda. Add the flour mixture, orange juice, and water to the sugar mixture; stir until well combined. Stir in the walnuts then distribute the mixture evenly into the mini muffin cups.

4 Bake for 15 to 18 minutes, or until a wooden toothpick inserted in the center comes out clean. Serve warm.

*To make this a gluten-free recipe, use nonstick cooking spray with no flour added, gluten-free vanilla extract, and seasoning with no added starch from a gluten-containing source. Substitute 1-1/2 cups rice flour plus 1/2 cup cornstarch for the all-purpose flour.

Exchanges
1 Carbohydrate

Calories 76
Calories from Fat . . . 22
Total Fat . . . . 2 g
Saturated Fat . . . . . . 0.7 g
Cholesterol . . . . 10 mg
Sodium . . . . 55 mg
Total Carbohydrate . . . 13 g
Dietary Fiber . . . . 1 g
Sugars . . . . 7 g
Protein . . . . 2 g

"Because we use whole-wheat flour instead of all-purpose flour, we've increased the amount of dietary fiber and lowered the calories in our mini muffins. Whole-wheat flour contains bran, so baked goods made with it are usually a little heavier and denser ... and better for us, too!"

Crunchy Oat-Apricot Bars

Serving Size: 1 bar; Total Servings: 36 bars

Nonstick cooking spray*

2 cups quick-cooking rolled oats*

1-3/4 cups all-purpose flour*

1 cup packed light brown sugar

1-1/2 teaspoons vanilla extract*

3/4 cup (1-1/2 sticks) light butter

1 jar (18 ounces) no-sugar-added apricot preserves

---

*To make this a gluten-free recipe, use nonstick cooking spray with no flour added, Irish oats, and gluten-free vanilla extract. Substitute 1-3/4 cups gluten-free flour blend plus 1/2 teaspoon xanthan gum for the all-purpose flour.

1 Preheat the oven to 350°F. Coat a 9" x 13" baking dish with non-stick cooking spray.

2 In a large bowl, combine the oats, flour, brown sugar, and vanilla extract. Cut the butter into the oat mixture with a pastry blender or 2 knives, until the mixture is crumbly.

3 Press half the oat mixture into the bottom of the baking dish. Spread the apricot preserves over the oat crust. Sprinkle the remaining oat mixture over the apricot preserves; press down gently.

4 Bake for 30 to 35 minutes, or until bubbly and golden. Cool completely in the baking dish on a wire rack. Cut into bars.

Exchanges
1 Carbohydrate
1/2 Fat

Calories 88
Calories from Fat . . . 21
Total Fat . . . . 2 g
Saturated Fat . . . . . . 1.4 g
Cholesterol . . . . 7 mg
Sodium . . . . 29 mg
Total Carbohydrate . . . 16 g
Dietary Fiber . . . . 1 g
Sugars . . . . 6 g
Protein . . . . 1 g

"The next time your kids tell you they need something for a bake sale, this is the perfect wholesome snack that everybody will love! Instead of baking tray after tray of drop cookies, try out this kid-friendly recipe that goes together in a jiffy."

Almond Cheesecake Tarts

Serving Size: 1 tart; Total Servings: 24

2 packages (8 ounces each) fat-free cream cheese, softened

1/2 cup plus 1 tablespoon sugar

3 eggs

1 teaspoon almond extract, divided*

1/2 teaspoon fresh lemon juice, divided

1 cup reduced-fat sour cream

1/4 cup slivered almonds

---

*To make this a gluten-free recipe, use gluten-free almond extract.

1 Preheat the oven to 325°F. Line mini muffin pans with foil muffin cup liners.

2 In a large bowl, combine the cream cheese and 1/2 cup sugar; beat well. Beat in the eggs one at a time then beat in 1/2 teaspoon almond extract and 1/4 teaspoon lemon juice until well combined. Spoon the mixture evenly into the muffin cups. Bake for 15 minutes.

3 Meanwhile, in a small bowl, combine the sour cream and the remaining 1 tablespoon sugar, 1/2 teaspoon almond extract, and 1/4 teaspoon lemon juice; mix well then spread over the cheesecake tarts. Top each with slivered almonds.

4 Bake for 10 minutes. Let cool, cover, and chill for at least 4 hours before serving.

Exchanges
1/2 Carbohydrate
1/2 Fat

Calories 63
  Calories from Fat . . . 19
Total Fat . . . . 2 g
  Saturated Fat . . . . . . 0.7 g
Cholesterol . . . . 32 mg
Sodium . . . . 115 mg
Total Carbohydrate . . . . 7 g
  Dietary Fiber . . . . 0 g
  Sugars . . . . 6 g
Protein . . . . 4 g

"If you love to bake, mini muffins can be your best friend because you can double and sometimes even triple a recipe by breaking it down into smaller portions. Remember, smaller portions are an important part of any meal plan. Plus, these tarts are so decadent, a smaller bite doesn't mean they're small on taste!"

Impossible Pumpkin Pie

Serving Size: 1 slice; Total Servings: 12

Nonstick cooking spray*

1 can (15 ounces) pure pumpkin

1 can (12 ounces) fat-free evaporated milk

1 tablespoon light butter, softened

2 eggs

1/2 cup sugar

1/2 cup reduced-fat biscuit baking mix*

2-1/2 teaspoons pumpkin pie spice*

2 teaspoons vanilla extract*

1 Preheat the oven to 350°F. Coat a 9-inch deep-dish pie plate with nonstick cooking spray.

2 Blend all the ingredients together in a blender on high speed for 1 minute, or place all the ingredients in a large bowl and beat for 2 minutes with a hand beater. Pour the mixture into the pie plate.

3 Bake for 50 to 60 minutes, or until a knife inserted in the center comes out clean.

4 Let cool then cover and chill for at least 2 hours before serving.

*To make this a gluten-free recipe, use nonstick cooking spray with no flour added, gluten-free biscuit mix and vanilla extract, and seasoning with no added starch from a gluten-containing source.

Exchanges
1 Carbohydrate
1/2 Fat

Calories 106
  Calories from Fat . . . 17
Total Fat . . . . 2 g
  Saturated Fat . . . . . . 0.7 g
Cholesterol . . . . 37 mg
Sodium . . . . 124 mg
Total Carbohydrate . . . 18 g
  Dietary Fiber . . . . 1 g
  Sugars . . . . 13 g
Protein . . . . 4 g

"Don't wait until Thanksgiving to serve up this new version of a classic holiday favorite. If you top each slice with a dollop of light whipped topping and a sprinkle of nutmeg, your family will be thanking you all year long!"

Crustless Lemon Cream Pie

Serving Size: 1 slice; Total Servings: 12

2 packages (4-serving-size each) sugar-free lemon gelatin

2 cups boiling water

1 cup ice cubes

2 cups frozen light whipped topping, thawed*

1 In a large bowl, dissolve the gelatin in the boiling water; add the ice cubes and stir until melted.

2 Add the whipped topping; mix until thoroughly combined. Pour into a 9-inch deep-dish pie plate.

3 Cover and chill for at least 3 hours, or until set.

*To make this a gluten-free recipe, use gluten-free whipped topping.

Exchanges
1/2 Fat

Calories 32
  Calories from Fat . . . 12
Total Fat . . . . 1 g
  Saturated Fat . . . . . . 1.3 g
Cholesterol . . . . 0 mg
Sodium . . . . 40 mg
Total Carbohydrate . . . . 3 g
  Dietary Fiber . . . . 0 g
  Sugars . . . . 1 g
Protein . . . . 1 g

"This isn't your ordinary fruit pie. No way! With the taste of tried-and-true lemon meringue pie, this treat is much simpler to make, and it's sure to work every time. You can use any flavor gelatin in here, so you're only limited by your imagination."

No-Bake Key Lime Pie

Serving Size: 1 slice; Total Servings: 12

Nonstick cooking spray*

1 package (4-serving-size)
sugar-free lime gelatin

1/2 cup boiling water

1 package (8 ounces) fat-free
cream cheese, softened

1 tablespoon fresh lime juice

1 teaspoon grated lime peel

2 cups frozen light whipped
topping, thawed*

1 Coat a 9-inch pie plate with
nonstick cooking spray.

2 In a small bowl, dissolve the gelatin in boiling water, stirring until
dissolved.

3 In a large bowl, beat the cream
cheese until smooth. Slowly add
the liquid gelatin until well
combined.

4 Stir in the lime juice and lime
peel. Fold in the whipped topping until well blended. Pour
into the pie plate, cover, and chill
for at least 3 hours, or until set.

*To make this a gluten-free recipe,
use nonstick cooking spray with no
flour added, and gluten-free whipped
topping.

Exchanges
1/2 Carbohydrate

Calories 46
  Calories from Fat . . . 12
Total Fat . . . . 1 g
  Saturated Fat . . . . . . 1.3 g
Cholesterol . . . . 2 mg
Sodium . . . . 122 mg
Total Carbohydrate . . . . 4 g
  Dietary Fiber . . . . 0 g
  Sugars . . . . 2 g
Protein . . . . 3 g

"Who doesn't love a no-bake dessert, especially when we're trying to keep the kitchen cool in summer? Just remember, as with any creamy dessert, if you're going to enjoy it outdoors, stay safe and keep it covered in the refrigerator or in a cooler, except during serving time. Don't let it stand before or after serving."

Orange Cream Pie

Serving Size: 1 slice; Total Servings: 12

1 container (8 ounces) fat-free frozen whipped topping, thawed

1 package (8 ounces) fat-free cream cheese, softened

1 teaspoon vanilla extract

1 package (4-serving-size) sugar-free orange gelatin

1 nine-inch reduced-fat graham cracker crust

1 In a medium bowl, cream together the whipped topping and cream cheese until smooth. Add the vanilla extract; beat until well combined. Sprinkle the gelatin mix over the top; stir until well combined.

2 Pour the orange cream mixture into the pie crust; cover and chill for at least two hours, or until set.

Exchanges
1 Carbohydrate
1/2 Fat

Calories 118
  Calories from Fat . . . 18
Total Fat . . . . 2 g
  Saturated Fat . . . . . . 0.7 g
Cholesterol . . . . 2 mg
Sodium . . . . 193 mg
Total Carbohydrate . . . 18 g
  Dietary Fiber . . . . 0 g
  Sugars . . . . 7 g
Protein . . . . 4 g

Options

Feel free to get creative and substitute your favorite kind of gelatin to make other kinds of creamy fruit-flavored pies.

Nicole's Banana Pudding Pie

Serving Size: 1 slice; Total Servings: 16

Nonstick cooking spray

1/2 of an 11-ounce box reduced-fat vanilla wafers

3 large ripe bananas, sliced

2 cups whole milk

1/3 cup plus 2 tablespoons sugar

2 tablespoons self-rising flour

1 teaspoon vanilla extract

1/8 teaspoon salt

2 eggs, separated

1 Preheat the oven to 400°F. Coat a deep-dish pie plate with nonstick cooking spray.

2 In the pie plate, layer half of the vanilla wafers then half of the sliced bananas. Repeat the layers one more time; set aside.

3 In a large saucepan, combine the milk, 1/3 cup sugar, the flour, vanilla extract, salt, and egg yolks. Cook over low heat until thickened, stirring constantly, about 10 minutes. Pour the cooked pudding mixture over the top of the banana layer in the pie plate.

4 Beat the egg whites until soft peaks form. Add the remaining 2 tablespoons sugar slowly to the egg whites and continue beating until stiff peaks form. Spread the meringue over the top of the pudding mixture.

5 Bake for 5 to 7 minutes, or until golden. Let cool then chill for at least 2 hours before serving.

Exchanges
1-1/2 Carbohydrate
1/2 Fat

Calories 118
Calories from Fat . . . 26
Total Fat . . . . 3 g
Saturated Fat . . . . . . 1.3 g
Cholesterol . . . . 29 mg
Sodium . . . . 71 mg
Total Carbohydrate . . . 21 g
Dietary Fiber . . . . 1 g
Sugars . . . . 15 g
Protein . . . . 2 g

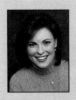

"When I'm ready to indulge in a well-deserved dessert, this banana pudding pie really hits the spot. Because there's less sugar in my version than in the traditional version of this normally super-sweet dessert, we're able to enjoy it just like everyone else."

Chocolate Almond Pavlova

Serving Size: 1 slice; Total Servings: 12

Nonstick cooking spray

3 egg whites, at room temperature

1/4 teaspoon cream of tartar

1/2 cup sugar

1/2 teaspoon vanilla extract

1 package (4-serving-size) sugar-free instant chocolate pudding mix

1-1/2 cups 1% milk

1/2 teaspoon almond extract

1 cup frozen light whipped topping, thawed

1 pint raspberries

1 Preheat the oven to 250°F. Coat a 9-inch deep-dish pie plate with nonstick cooking spray.

2 In a large bowl, beat the egg whites and cream of tartar with an electric mixer on high speed for 5 minutes, or until soft peaks form. Add the sugar and beat until stiff peaks form.

3 Fold in the vanilla extract then spoon the mixture into the pie plate, spreading the meringue evenly over the bottom and up the sides of the plate.

4 Bake for 1 hour, or until light golden; let cool.

5 In a medium bowl, combine the pudding mix, milk, and almond extract; beat until slightly thickened. Fold in the whipped topping then pour mixture into the cooled meringue crust. Top with the raspberries and serve, or chill until ready to serve.

Exchanges
1 Carbohydrate

Calories 81
Calories from Fat . . . 10
Total Fat . . . . 1 g
Saturated Fat . . . . . . 0.9 g
Cholesterol . . . . 2 mg
Sodium . . . . 140 mg
Total Carbohydrate . . . 15 g
Dietary Fiber . . . . 1 g
Sugars . . . . 11 g
Protein . . . . 2 g

Did You Know . . .

that Pavlova, a soft meringue cake, is a traditional Australian dessert named after the Russian ballerina Anna Pavlova? This beautiful cake has a meringue crust filled with whipped topping, custard, or pudding. Sliced strawberries, kiwi, or other fresh fruit look terrific on top.

Tart Bubblin' Blueberry Crisp

Serving Size: 1/2 cup; Total Servings: 8

Nonstick cooking spray*

2 pints (16 ounces) fresh blueberries

1/4 cup plus 2 tablespoons all-purpose flour, divided*

2 tablespoons granulated sugar

1/2 teaspoon ground cinnamon*

1/2 cup quick-cooking rolled oats*

3 tablespoons light brown sugar

2 tablespoons reduced-fat stick margarine, softened

---

*To make this a gluten-free recipe, use nonstick cooking spray with no flour added, 1/4 cup tapioca flour plus 2 tablespoons potato starch flour instead of all-purpose flour, seasoning with no added starch from a gluten-containing source, and Irish oats.

1 Preheat the oven to 400°F. Coat a 9-inch microwave-safe pie plate with nonstick cooking spray.

2 In a large bowl, combine the blueberries, 2 tablespoons flour, the granulated sugar, and cinnamon; mix well. Spoon into the pie plate and cover with wax paper. Microwave on high power for 4 to 5 minutes, or until the berries are bubbly.

3 Meanwhile, in a medium bowl, combine the remaining 1/4 cup flour, oats, and brown sugar; mix well. With a fork, blend in the margarine until crumbly. Sprinkle the mixture over the blueberries.

4 Bake in the oven for 12 to 15 minutes, or until the top is golden. Serve warm.

Exchanges
1-1/2 Carbohydrate
1/2 Fat

Calories 125
  Calories from Fat . . . 18
Total Fat . . . . 2 g
  Saturated Fat . . . . . . 0.3 g
Cholesterol . . . . 0 mg
Sodium . . . . 25 mg
Total Carbohydrate . . . 26 g
  Dietary Fiber . . . . 3 g
  Sugars . . . . 14 g
Protein . . . . 2 g

"Blueberries contain compounds that may help reduce the risk of certain cancers and cardiovascular and other diseases, so it's important to include them in a healthy meal plan. Aside from blueberries, raspberries, peaches, blackberries, and other fruit all work great in dessert crisps, so use whatever's in season and reap the benefits!"

Nutty Baked Apples

Serving Size: 1 apple half; Total Servings: 8

4 medium baking apples

2 cups water

1 cinnamon stick

1/3 cup chopped walnuts

2 tablespoons light butter, melted

2 tablespoons light brown sugar

3/4 teaspoon ground cinnamon, divided*

1/4 teaspoon ground nutmeg*

1 tablespoon granulated sugar

---

*To make this a gluten-free recipe, use seasonings with no added starch from a gluten-containing source.

1 Preheat the oven to 375°F.

2 Cut the apples in half horizontally and core them (see Tip), making sure not to go through the bottoms. Place the apples cut-side up in a 9" x 13" baking dish. Pour water around the apples and place the cinnamon stick in the water.

3 In a small bowl, combine the walnuts, butter, brown sugar, 1/2 teaspoon cinnamon, and nutmeg; mix well. Stuff the mixture evenly into the apples.

4 In another small bowl, combine the remaining 1/4 teaspoon cinnamon and the granulated sugar; sprinkle evenly over the apples.

5 Cover the baking dish tightly with aluminum foil. Bake for 30 to 35 minutes, or until the apples are tender. Serve warm.

Exchanges
1 Carbohydrate
1 Fat

Calories	100
Calories from Fat	44
Total Fat	5 g
Saturated Fat	1.3 g
Cholesterol	5 mg
Sodium	22 mg
Total Carbohydrate	15 g
Dietary Fiber	2 g
Sugars	12 g
Protein	1 g

Preparation Tip

If you don't have an apple corer, you can use a melon baller, a spoon, or knife—just make sure not to go through the bottom of the apples.

Chocolate Peanut Butter Trifle

Serving Size: 1 square; Total Servings: 12

1 package (4-serving-size) sugar-free instant chocolate pudding mix

2 cups fat-free milk

1 container (8 ounces) fat-free frozen whipped topping, thawed, divided

1/2 cup reduced-fat peanut butter

1/2 of a store-bought angel food cake, cut into 1/2-inch slices

2 tablespoons chopped peanuts

1 In a large bowl, beat the pudding mix and milk until well combined. Place 1 cup pudding in a medium bowl, reserving the remaining pudding. Add 1 cup whipped topping to the 1 cup pudding; fold until well blended.

2 In another medium bowl, beat the peanut butter into the remaining whipped topping until smooth.

3 Line the bottom of an 8-inch square baking dish with half of the angel food cake slices. Spread the chocolate whipped topping mixture evenly over the cake slices, followed by a second layer of the remaining angel food cake slices then a layer of chocolate pudding. Spread the peanut butter mixture over the pudding.

4 Sprinkle with the chopped peanuts. Cover and chill for at least 1 hour before serving.

Exchanges
2 Carbohydrate
1 Fat

Calories	198
Calories from Fat	41
Total Fat	5 g
Saturated Fat	1.0 g
Cholesterol	1 mg
Sodium	174 mg
Total Carbohydrate	32 g
Dietary Fiber	2 g
Sugars	15 g
Protein	7 g

Serving Tip

If you're looking for the ultimate dessert presentation, make these in parfait glasses so the decadent layers can win you loads of raves!

Peach Melba 'n' Cream Squares

Serving Size: 1 square; Total Servings: 9

1 package (10 ounces) frozen peach slices, thawed

1/2 of an 11-ounce box reduced-fat vanilla wafers, coarsely crushed

1 container (8 ounces) fat-free frozen whipped topping, thawed

3/4 cup sugar-free raspberry preserves, melted

1/4 cup fresh raspberries

1 Place one-third of the peaches on the bottom of an 8-inch square baking dish. Top with one-third of the crushed wafers and one-third of the whipped topping then drizzle with one-third of the raspberry preserves. Repeat the layers two more times.

2 Garnish with fresh raspberries and serve, or cover and chill until ready to serve.

Exchanges

2 Carbohydrate

Calories 143
  Calories from Fat . . . 19
Total Fat . . . . 2 g
  Saturated Fat . . . . . . 0.9 g
Cholesterol . . . . 0 mg
Sodium . . . . 46 mg
Total Carbohydrate . . . 28 g
  Dietary Fiber . . . . 1 g
  Sugars . . . . 13 g
Protein . . . . 1 g

"This crowd-pleaser can't possibly get any easier to make. It doesn't matter how busy you are, this no-bake classic is a simple yet elegant dessert that tastes as good as it looks! Just wait 'til you see their eyes light up when you place this on the dinner table!"

Pecan Pear Squares

Serving Size: 1 square; Total Servings: 20

Nonstick cooking spray*

2-1/4 cups all-purpose flour*

1 cup packed light brown sugar

1/4 cup (1/2 stick) light butter, softened

1 can (15 ounces) pears in light syrup, chopped, juice reserved

1/2 cup egg substitute

1 teaspoon vanilla extract*

2 teaspoons baking soda

1 teaspoon salt

3 tablespoons chopped pecans

1 Preheat the oven to 350°F. Coat a 9" x 13" baking dish with non-stick cooking spray.

2 In a large bowl, using an electric mixer, beat the flour, brown sugar, butter, reserved pear juice, egg substitute, vanilla extract, baking soda, and salt for 2 minutes or until smooth. Stir in the chopped pears then pour the mixture into the baking dish; top with the chopped pecans.

3 Bake for 25 to 30 minutes, or until a wooden toothpick inserted in the center comes out clean. Allow to cool completely then cut into squares and serve, or store in an airtight container until ready to serve.

*To make this a gluten-free recipe, use nonstick cooking spray with no flour added, and vanilla extract with no added starch from a gluten-containing source. Substitute 1 cup gluten-free flour blend plus 1/4 teaspoon xanthan gum for the all-purpose flour.

Exchanges
1-1/2 Carbohydrate
1/2 Fat

Calories	124
Calories from Fat	20
Total Fat	2 g
Saturated Fat	0.9 g
Cholesterol	4 mg
Sodium	274 mg
Total Carbohydrate	24 g
Dietary Fiber	1 g
Sugars	13 g
Protein	2 g

Good For You

Would you believe that a handful of pecans (one ounce) contains only 4 grams of carbohydrates? Yup, pecans are so good for us that we can use them to top our salads or crust our fish, chicken, and pork. We can eat them as a snack or add 'em to our desserts ... guilt-free!

Fruit Squares

Serving Size: 1 square; Total Servings: 9

2 cups no-sugar-added applesauce

2 packages (4-serving-size) sugar-free strawberry gelatin

1 cup crushed pineapple in its own juice

1 can (12 ounces) diet lemon-lime soda (1-3/4 cups)

1 In a medium saucepan, bring the applesauce to a boil over medium-high heat. Remove from the heat and add the gelatin, pineapple, and soda; mix well then pour into an 8-inch square baking dish.

2 Let cool then cover and chill for at least 3 hours, or until set. Cut into squares and serve.

Thumbs-up for gluten-free meal plans!

Exchanges
1/2 Fruit

Calories	44
Calories from Fat	0
Total Fat	0 g
Saturated Fat	0.0 g
Cholesterol	0 mg
Sodium	55 mg
Total Carbohydrate	10 g
Dietary Fiber	1 g
Sugars	8 g
Protein	1 g

"If you're still trying to find ways to get your kids (and those young at heart) to eat more fruit, here's a fun way to tempt their taste buds! Different fruits and sugar-free fruit gelatins combine to make a tasty duo that's a great alternative to high-calorie, packaged snacks."

Caramel Espresso Brownies

Serving Size: 1 square; Total Servings: 16

Nonstick cooking spray*

1 tablespoon instant coffee granules

2 tablespoons water

2/3 cup all-purpose flour*

2/3 cup sugar

1/2 cup unsweetened cocoa

1/4 cup (1/2 stick) light butter, melted

1/3 cup egg substitute

1 teaspoon vanilla extract*

1/2 teaspoon baking powder

1/4 cup caramel sauce*

1 Preheat the oven to 350°F. Coat an 8-inch square baking dish with nonstick cooking spray.

2 In a large bowl, dissolve the coffee granules in the water. Add the remaining ingredients except the caramel sauce; mix well. Pour the batter into the baking dish. Drizzle with caramel sauce and, using a knife, swirl the sauce into the batter.

3 Bake for 25 to 30 minutes, or until a wooden toothpick inserted in the center comes out clean. Let cool completely. Cut into squares and serve, or store in an airtight container until ready to serve.

*To make this a gluten-free recipe, use nonstick cooking spray with no flour added, and gluten-free vanilla extract and caramel sauce. Substitute 2/3 cup minus 2 tablespoons brown rice flour for the all-purpose flour.

Exchanges

1 Carbohydrate
1/2 Fat

Calories 89
  Calories from Fat . . . 17
Total Fat . . . . 2 g
  Saturated Fat . . . . . . 1.1 g
Cholesterol . . . . 4 mg
Sodium . . . . 59 mg
Total Carbohydrate . . . 18 g
  Dietary Fiber . . . . 1 g
  Sugars . . . . 11 g
Protein . . . . 2 g

Finishing Touch

To give these brownies a fancy flair, serve each with a sprinkle of confectioners' sugar and a sprig of fresh mint.

Peach Melba Parfaits

Serving Size: 1 parfait; Total Servings: 6

1 package (10 ounces) frozen peach slices, thawed

2 tablespoons reduced-fat butter, thinly sliced

3 tablespoons light brown sugar

1 pint fat-free vanilla frozen yogurt*

1/2 pint fresh raspberries

1 bunch fresh mint (optional)

See photo insert following page 84.

1 In a small saucepan, combine the peaches, butter, and brown sugar. Cook over low heat until the butter is melted and the sugar is dissolved.

2 Scoop the frozen yogurt evenly into individual serving bowls or parfait glasses then spoon the peach mixture over the top.

3 Garnish with the fresh raspberries and mint sprigs, if desired.

*To make this a gluten-free recipe, use gluten-free frozen yogurt.

Exchanges
1-1/2 Carbohydrate
1/2 Fat

Calories 130
  Calories from Fat . . . 19
Total Fat . . . . 2 g
  Saturated Fat . . . . . . 1.2 g
Cholesterol . . . . 5 mg
Sodium . . . . 64 mg
Total Carbohydrate . . . 26 g
  Dietary Fiber . . . . 2 g
  Sugars . . . . 20 g
Protein . . . . 3 g

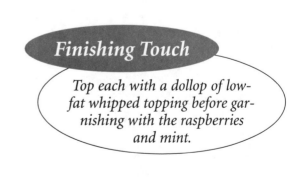

Finishing Touch

Top each with a dollop of low-fat whipped topping before garnishing with the raspberries and mint.

Fresh Mango Sorbet

Serving Size: 1/3 cup; Total Servings: 6

2 ripe mangos

1 cup Splenda

3/4 cup water

Juice of 1 lime

1 Peel the mangos and cut as much of the fruit away from the pits as possible; discard the skin and pits.

2 Place the mango flesh and the remaining ingredients in a food processor or blender; blend until completely smooth. Pour into an ice cube tray; cover and freeze overnight.

3 Remove frozen mango mixture from the tray and process in a food processor until smooth. Serve, or cover and freeze until ready to serve.

Thumbs-up for gluten-free meal plans!

Exchanges
1 Fruit

Calories 62
   Calories from Fat 2
Total Fat . . . . 0 g
   Saturated Fat . . . . . . 0.0 g
Cholesterol . . . . 0 mg
Sodium . . . . 2 mg
Total Carbohydrate . . . 16 g
   Dietary Fiber . . . . 1 g
   Sugars . . . . 14 g
Protein . . . . 0 g

Did You Know . . .

that the artificial sweetener Splenda can be added directly to foods and that it works well for cooking and baking too?

Lemon Italian Ice

Serving Size: 1/3 cup; Total Servings: 9

2 cups water

3/4 cup fresh lemon juice

3/4 cup sugar

2 teaspoons grated lemon peel

1 In a medium saucepan, combine all the ingredients. Bring to a boil over medium heat, stirring constantly. Remove from the heat and allow to cool for 5 minutes.

2 Pour the mixture into 2 ice cube trays. Cover and freeze overnight.

3 Remove frozen mixture from the trays and pulse in a food processor or blender for 2 to 3 minutes, or until the consistency is thick and creamy. Serve, or cover and freeze until ready to serve.

Thumbs-up for gluten-free meal plans!

Exchanges
1 Carbohydrate

Calories 66
  Calories from Fat 1
Total Fat . . . . 0 g
  Saturated Fat . . . . . . 0.0 g
Cholesterol . . . . 0 mg
Sodium . . . . 4 mg
Total Carbohydrate . . . 17 g
  Dietary Fiber . . . . 0 g
  Sugars . . . . 17 g
Protein . . . . 0 g

"Because we keep this frozen, we can pull it out whenever we need a refreshing snack. Serve it up at your next backyard bash, poolside, or as a light after-school or anytime pick-me-up."

Sugar-Free Gummy Worms

Serving Size: 1 "worm"; Total Servings: 28

Nonstick cooking spray*

2 packages (4-serving-size) sugar-free gelatin (any flavor)

2 envelopes (1/3 ounce each) unsweetened soft drink mix* (any flavor)

3 envelopes (1 ounce each) unflavored gelatin

1 cup boiling water

1 Coat an 8-inch square baking dish with nonstick cooking spray.

2 In a medium bowl, combine all the ingredients until dissolved. Pour into the baking dish, cover, and chill for 2 to 3 hours, or until completely set.

3 Cut into 1/4-inch strips to form thin "worms" for serving as is or decorating other treats.

*To make this a gluten-free recipe, use nonstick cooking spray with no flour added, and gluten-free soft drink mix.

Exchanges
Free food

Calories 14
   Calories from Fat 0
Total Fat . . . . 0 g
   Saturated Fat . . . . . . 0.0 g
Cholesterol . . . . 0 mg
Sodium . . . . 23 mg
Total Carbohydrate . . . . 1 g
   Dietary Fiber . . . . 0 g
   Sugars . . . . 0 g
Protein . . . . 3 g

Preparation Tip

If you're a real candy connoisseur, you might want to make these in fun candy molds for fancier gummy candy.

Alphabetical List of Recipes

Subject Index

About the American Diabetes Association

The American Diabetes Association is the nation's leading voluntary health organization supporting diabetes research, information, and advocacy. Its mission is to prevent and cure diabetes and to improve the lives of all people affected by diabetes. The American Diabetes Association is the leading publisher of comprehensive diabetes information. Its huge library of practical and authoritative books for people with diabetes covers every aspect of self-care—cooking and nutrition, fitness, weight control, medications, complications, emotional issues, and general self-care.

To order American Diabetes Association books: Call 1-800-232-6733 or log on to http://store.diabetes.org.

To join the American Diabetes Association: Call 1-800-806-7801 or log on to www.diabetes.org/membership.

For more information about diabetes or ADA programs and services: Call 1-800-342-2383. E-mail: AskADA@diabetes.org or log on to www.diabetes.org.

To locate an ADA/NCQA Recognized Provider of quality diabetes care in your area: www.ncqa.org/dprp

To find an ADA Recognized Education Program in your area: Call 1-800-342-2383. www.diabetes.org/for-health-professionals-and-scientists/recognition/edrecognition.jsp

To join the fight to increase funding for diabetes research, end discrimination, and improve insurance coverage: Call 1-800-342-2383. www.diabetes.org/advocacy-and-legalresources/advocacy.jsp

To find out how you can get involved with the programs in your community: Call 1-800-342-2383. See below for program Web addresses.

- *American Diabetes Month:* educational activities for people diagnosed with diabetes; occurs in November. www.diabetes.org/communityprograms-and-localevents/americandiabetesmonth.jsp
- *American Diabetes Alert:* annual public awareness campaign to find the undiagnosed; held the fourth Tuesday in March. www.diabetes.org/communityprograms-and-localevents/americandiabetesalert.jsp
- *The Diabetes Assistance & Resources Program (DAR):* diabetes awareness program targeted to the Latino community. www.diabetes.org/communityprograms-and-localevents/latinos.jsp
- *African American Program:* diabetes awareness program targeted to the African American community. www.diabetes.org/communityprograms-and-localevents/africanamericans.jsp
- *Awakening the Spirit: Pathways to Diabetes Prevention & Control:* diabetes awareness program targeted to the Native American community. www.diabetes.org/communityprograms-and-localevents/nativeamericans.jsp

To find out about an important research project regarding type 2 diabetes: www.diabetes.org/diabetes-research/research-home.jsp

To obtain information on making a planned gift or charitable bequest: Call 1-888-700-7029. www.wpg.cc/stl/CDA/homepage/1,1006,509,00.html

To make a donation or memorial contribution: Call 1-800-342-2383. www.diabetes.org/support-the-cause/make-a-donation.jsp